Mama's Menu

Ayurvedic Recipes for Postpartum Healing

By Ameya Duprey

Disclaimer

This book is not intended to treat, diagnose or prescribe. The information contained herein is in no way meant to be a substitute for a duly licensed health care professional.

COPYRIGHT © 2020 BY AMY DUPREY

First Edition, 2020

Acknowledgements

Editors: Bandhu Gulbis and Sarai Devi Dasi
Cover Illustration: Sarai Devi Dasi
Foreword: Alakananda Ma
Photography: Sarai Devi Dasi
Photography Equipment: Akhi Lavoie
Vedic Astrology: Kari Field

Dedication

To My Teachers

My mother June ~ *who inspired the joy of cooking within me.*

Alakananda Ma ~ *who took me under her wing as a youthful seeker and taught me many things including Ayurveda, vegetarian cooking, Sanatana Dharma and ashram life.*

Ysha Oakes ~ *without whom this book would not exist. May her legacy of teaching Ayurvedic postpartum care be carried on into the future, and her soul be bathed in Eternal Bliss.*

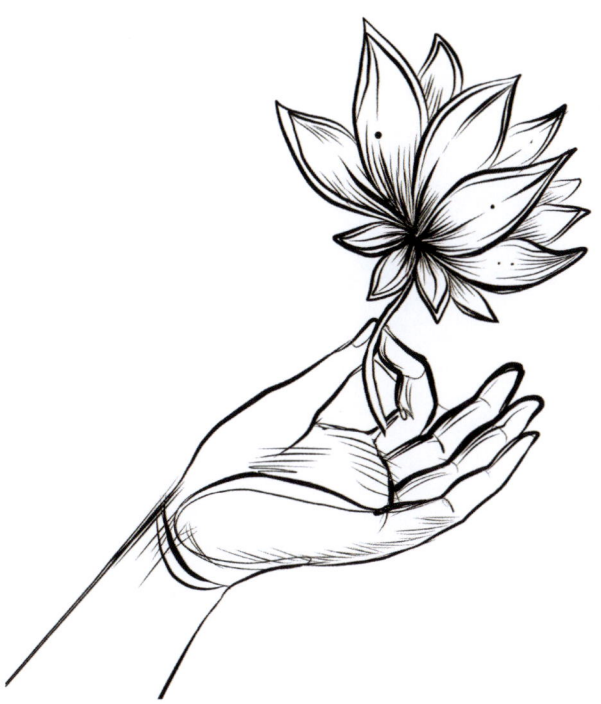

Table of Contents

Foreward 8

Introduction 9

Part 1: Food as Medicine

Chapter 1: Ayurveda 101   12

    The 5 Elements 13

    The 3 Constitutions of Ayurveda 14

    The 20 Physical Qualities of Creation 16

    The 3 Subtle Qualities of Creation 17

Chapter 2: The Ayurvedic Postpartum Diet   19

    Ayurvedic Diet Energetics 20

    Cultivating Strong Digestion After Birth 21

    Food Combining 22

    Cultivating Vitality Through Proper Diet 23

    Healing Postpartum Foods 24

    Foods to Avoid After Birth 25

    The 4 Phases of an Ayurvedic Postpartum Diet 25

    Transitioning Back to a Regular Diet 26

    Rebalancing After Birth 27

Chapter 3: Getting Prepared   29

    Kitchen Tools 30

    Mama's Menu Grocery List 31

    Where to Find Unfamiliar Ingredients 33

Part 2: Recipes for Postpartum Healing

Chapter 1: Days 1-3 ~Foundational Recipes   35

    Strong Fenugreek Tea 36

First Days Rice Congee 37

Mother's Milk 38

Vital Garlic Chutney 39

Raab 40

Cream of Rice Cereal with Dates 41

Healing Mung Dal Soup 42

Calming Kitchari 43

Almond Kheer 44

Crustless Apple Pie 45

Mama's Masala 46

Ghee 47

Chapter 2: Days 4-10 ~ Digestion and Lactation   48

Simple Lactation Tea 49

Mother's Red Chai 50

Iron-Rich Smoothie 51

Sweet & Simple Tahini Milk 52

La Horchata de Mamá 53

RejuvenDate Shake 54

Cream of Wheat with Ground Almonds 55

Coconut Maple Tapioca Pudding 56

Replenishing Urad Dal Soup 57

Womb Rejuvenating Kitchari 58

Mama's Mung Soup 59

Chai Spice Kitchari with Fennel 60

Iron-Rich Tamarind Chutney 61

Tasty Quinoa 62

Simple Postpartum Rice 63

Butternut Squash Soup 64

Daughter's Delight Cardamom Cream 65

Divine Caramel Halva 66

Cardamom Vanilla Rice Pudding 67

Yam Halva 68

Sesame Halva 69

Soothing Pear Delight 70

Chapter 3: Days 11-21 ~ Lactation and Rejuvination   71

Strawberry & Cream Smoothie 72

Oatmeal with Crystalized Ginger 73

Hearty Roots & Barley Stew 74

Creamy Beet Soup with Tarragon 75

Hearty Mung Bean Soup 76

Vegetable Coconut Curry 77

Sweet Potatoes and Greens 78

Curried Beets 79

Sweet Potato Mash 80

Happy Baby Fennel Dish 81

Glazed Carrots 82

Gingered Greens 83

Fresh Paneer Cheese 84

Sag Paneer 85

Vegan Lactation Pesto 86

Mother's Guacamole 87

Avocado Chutney with Crystalized Ginger 88

Cumin Chapati Flatbread 89

Garlic Farinata 90

Snacking Almonds 91

Mother's Mexican Wedding Cookies 92

Iron-Rich Ginger Cookies 93

Chapter 4: Days 22-42 ~ Rejuvenation   **94**

Sesame Ginger-Snap Amaranth 95

Toor Dal with Pumpkin 96

Black Bean Soup 97

Oh Baby "Baked" Beans 98

Pesto Sweet Potato Fries 99

Channa Dal Hummus 100

Garden Pasta with Pesto and Cheese 101

Delicious Yam Patties 102

Coconut Mint Chutney 103

Black Bean Croquets 104

Vegetable Koorma with Fennel 105

Curried Black Bean and Sweet Potato Burrito 106

Postnatal Pad Thai 107

Fig Crescents 108

Foreword

Over the last thirty years of practicing Ayurveda, all too often I have heard the same story: "My health was fine until the birth of my first/second/third child." Maternal depletion syndrome or postpartum depletion are terms that have been coined to describe a state of general depletion following the demands of pregnancy and lactation. It may be challenging for a woman to return to optimum health, especially amid the many demands of contemporary lifestyles.

A mother herself, Ameya has taken to heart the needs of new mothers. In Mama's Menu, she shares recipes and a holistic approach that will help provide the best possible outcomes for you, as a new mother. In addition, you will learn some of the basic Ayurvedic teachings regarding food, diet and digestion. This will empower you to take charge of your own and your family's diet as you transition back to a regular diet. I am sure many of these delicious recipes will continue to be a part of your ongoing menu plan!

Alakananda Ma
Alandi Ayurveda Clinic
July 2020

Introduction

When you birth a child into this world, it is not only your baby who gets a fresh start in life. Life automatically hits the reset button for you as well, as you are reborn into a mother's body. Channeling the force of creation is a very powerful act and uses an immense amount of energy. Whether you are ready or not, you will have to start from square one to regain your vitality. For the first six weeks after birth, it is essential for you to focus not only on your newborn's needs, but also on your own rejuvenation.

One of the most important aspects of postpartum recovery is diet. Hippocrates, the father of modern medicine, said, "Let food be thy medicine." Unfortunately, western medicine does not offer much insight into the practicals of food as medicine. Ayurveda, on the other hand, focuses on the qualities of the food we eat as the primary input into our state of health. Your postpartum diet will not only affect the quality of your recovery, but also the quality of the breast milk you feed your baby. Having a healthy postpartum diet is essential for your own healing, as well as your baby's nourishment.

So what's the best postpartum diet?

Here in America, one luxury that we don't have is traditional postpartum wisdom. Because of this, we must look towards other cultures and traditions for guidance on postpartum care and diet.

Ayurveda, literally meaning "the wisdom of life," is a holistic system of healthcare that has been practiced in India for over 5,000 years. Unlike the West, which focuses almost completely on prenatal care, Ayurveda offers a complete system with more focus on postnatal care, in which a specialized postpartum diet plays the central role.

As an Ayurvedic postpartum doula, I cannot stress enough how impactful your diet is on your postpartum recovery. It effects everything: your quality of sleep, bowel movements, energy level, digestion, moods, and recovery time as well as your baby's comfort and digestion. So many unnecessary stresses can be avoided if you simply know what to eat!

If it's really that simple, then why don't more people know about it?

I ask myself this question all the time. Ayurveda is still relatively new in America, and so is the practice of postpartum care. There are still very few practitioners who carry this knowledge here in the West. It is beyond time for mothers to get the care they need to regain their vitality after birth.

Drawing from my background in Ayurvedic vegetarian cooking and postpartum care, I have created this cookbook as a tool for postnatal self-healing. The recipes in Mama's Menu ensure that you are receiving the best foods to nourish and revitalize your body during this unique time in your life. With Mama's Menu at your fingertips, you will be well on your way to regaining your strength and vitality.

It is my sincere desire to see the rise of postpartum care practices here in the West. I pray that this book will help countless mothers regain their vitality and rest in bliss with their babies. You absolutely deserve it.

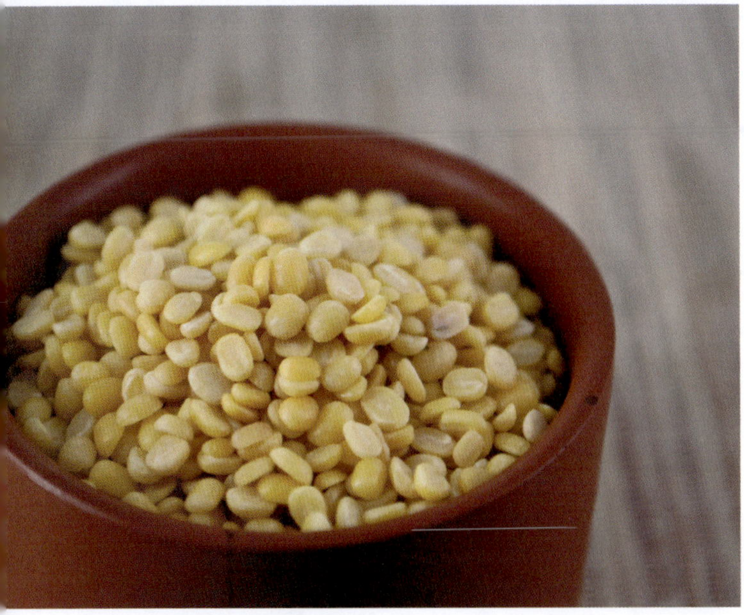

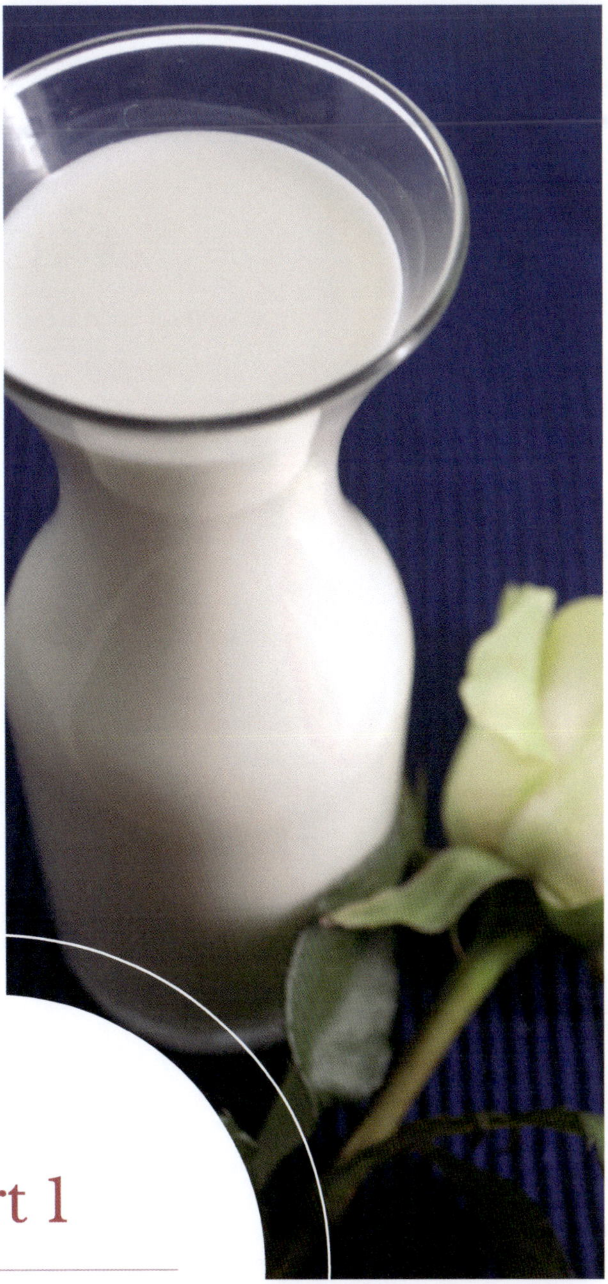

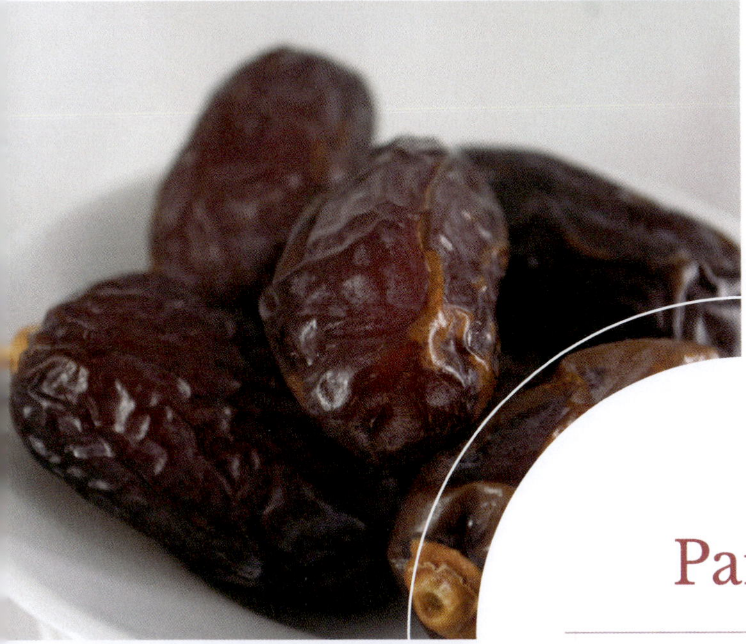

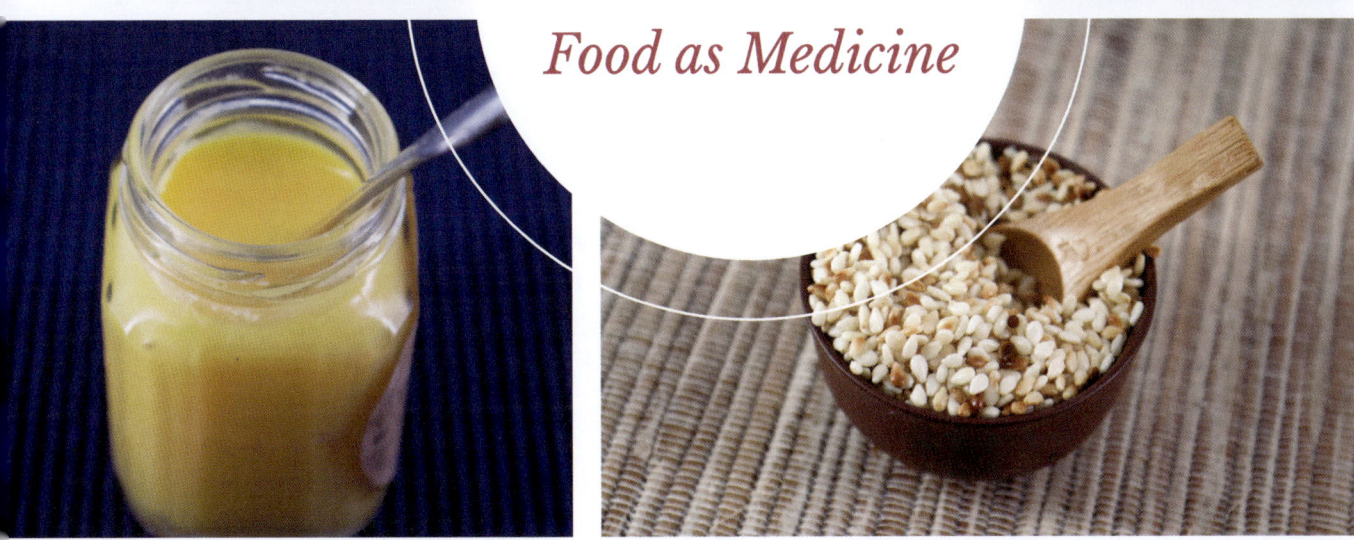

Part 1

Food as Medicine

Chapter 1
Ayurveda 101

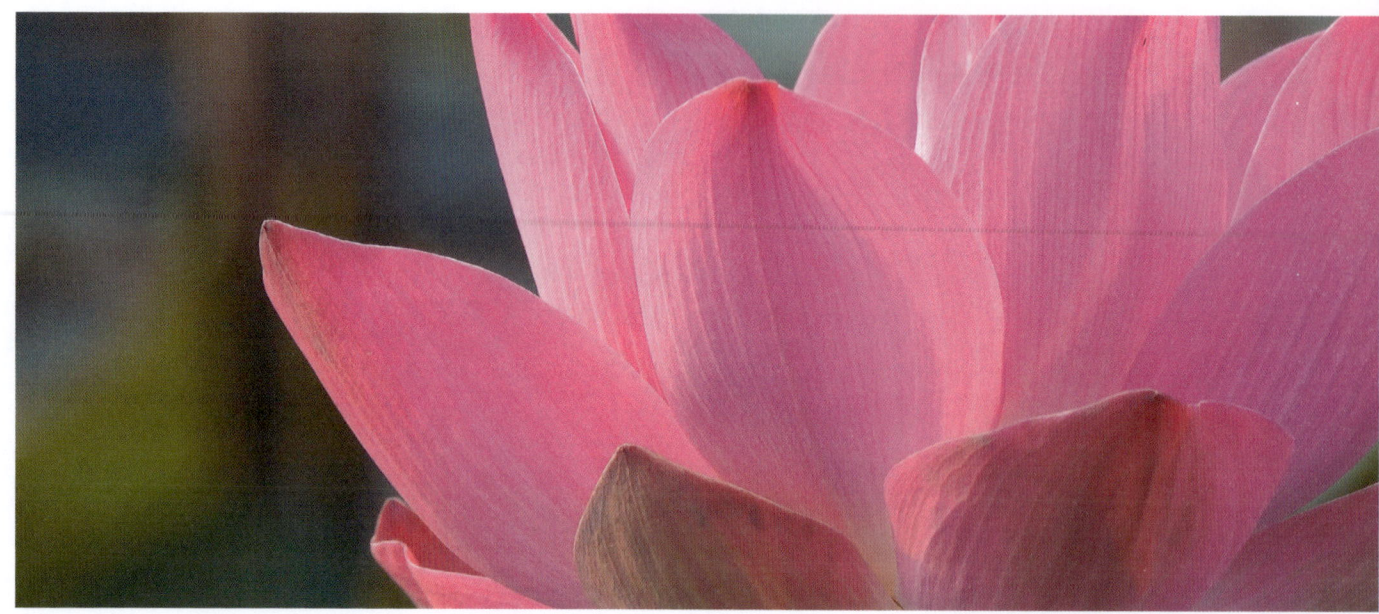

Ayurveda is a holistic system of healthcare that has been practiced in India for thousands of years. Ayurvedic medicine brings balance and healing to all aspects of daily living through diet, lifestyle, herbal medicine, cleansing, and rejuvenation therapies.

In order to find balance within our bodies and mind, we must first know the forces at play that are affecting our lives and our health. In this chapter you will learn basic Ayurvedic concepts and how they apply to your postnatal diet and health. We will explore the 5 elements, 3 constitutional types, 20 physical qualities and 3 subtle qualities of creation.

The 5 Elements

All of physical existence is made up of these 5 elements:

Ether   Air   Fire   Water   Earth

Ether, or Space, is the basis from which all the other elements manifest. Space provides the room for everything in creation to happen. Ether manifests in our bodies as the empty spaces such as our bladder, stomach, lungs, and in women, our womb. After birth, this element becomes imbalanced with the large empty space created by the sudden exit of the baby from the uterus.

The second element, Air, moves like the wind. It is restless, quick and ever-changing. Air is ether in action. Air manifests in our bodies as the movements that initiate all bodily functions. The movement of the air element increases to birth your baby, and will need to be rebalanced postpartum.

Fire is the third element, which is the transformative energy in creation. Within our bodies, it is the force that allows us to digest and assimilate food as well as experiences. Fire is the light in our eyes, the brightness of our minds and the digestive power in our bellies. This fire element of digestion becomes imbalanced after birth by burning so much transformative energy to birth your baby.

Water is life. It is the fourth element and nurtures all of creation. Within our bodies it is our blood, lymph, saliva, digestive juices, and in women, our breast milk. Due to the loss of fluids from birthing as well as breastfeeding, our water element becomes diminished and will need extra fluids and oils to be rebalanced.

The fifth element, Earth, is the grounding force on which we live. It supports our bodies, homes and food. It provides the foundation for our physical existence. Within our bodies it gives us our structural foundation, our skeleton. The grounding force of earth is what our bodies need most after birth. Food inherently contains an abundance of the earth element. With proper guidance in postnatal nutrition, the food you eat will be a great medicine for your postpartum rejuvenation.

The 3 Constitutions of Ayurveda

One of the foundational principles of Ayurveda is the 3 constitutional types, or *doshas*: *vata*, *pitta* and *kapha*. Each dosha is made of varying combinations of the 5 elements: space, fire, air, water and earth. *Vata* is a mixture of space and air. *Pitta* is fire with a splash of water. *Kapha* is a combination of water and earth. All 3 constitutions have their own inherent attributes, as seen below:

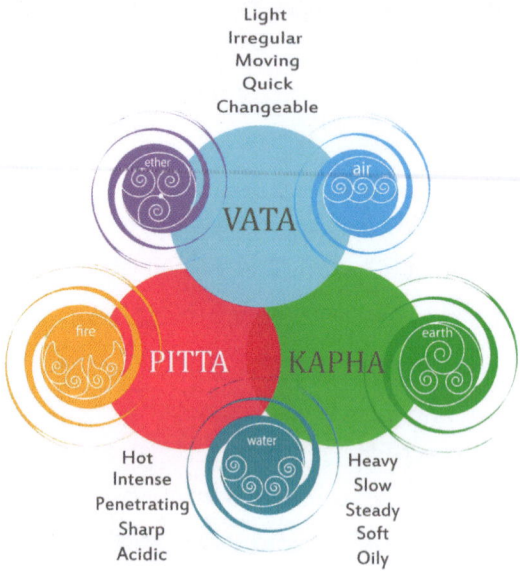

All 3 constitutional types live within us to varying degrees. We are each born with a unique constitutional fingerprint that remains the same throughout our entire lives. The constitutional type that is predominant at birth and throughout our lives is called our *prakriti*. It could be vata, pitta or kapha. You can even have two predominant constitutions such as vata-pitta, pitta-kapha and occasionally vata-kapha.

When we aggravate our innate constitution through our thoughts, actions or environment, our natural balance is thrown off. These imbalances are called *vikruti*, and allow diseases to manifest inside our bodies. Having a baby throws vata out of balance. If you ignore this imbalance, it can become deep-seated and manifest as chronic illness later on down the road.

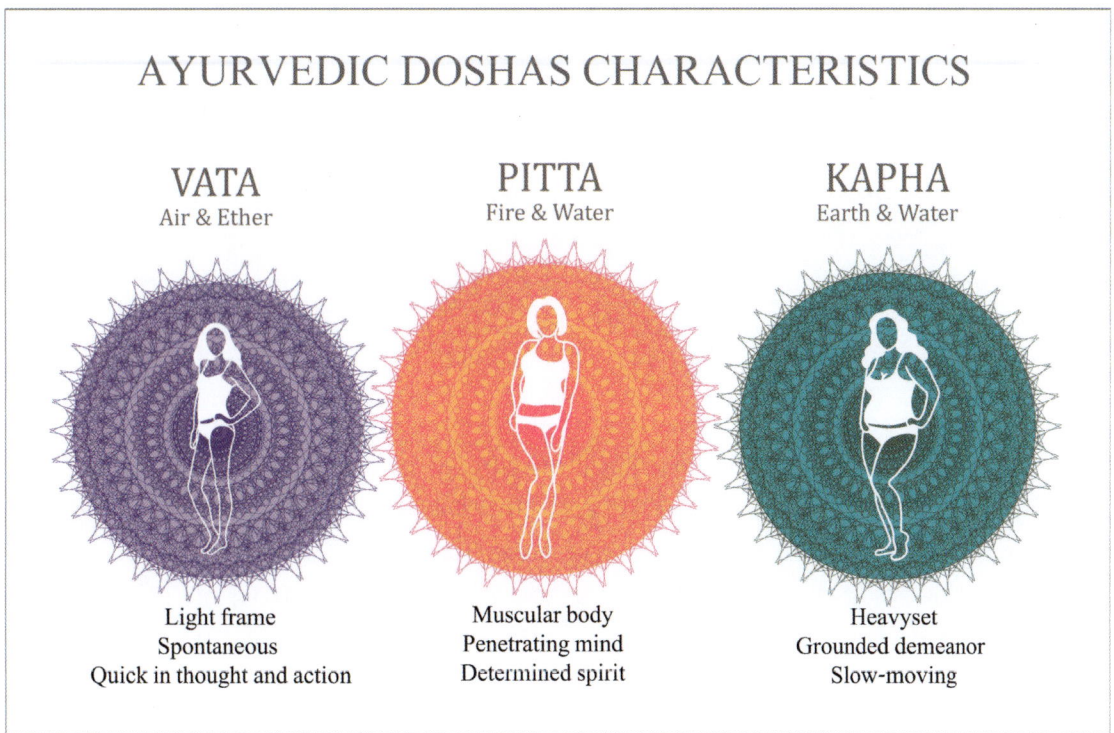

Below you will find a simple description of each constitutional type (dosha) and how it relates to our bodies, mind, emotions and experiences.

Vata by nature is wind and movement. It regulates all activity in the body. When in balance it promotes creativity and flexibility and evokes feelings of freshness, lightness, happiness and joy. When out of balance it evokes fear, anxiety, worry, nervousness, tremors and spasms.

Pitta is the principle of fire, warmth and digestion. When in balance it promotes intelligence and understanding. When out of balance it evokes anger, hatred, jealousy and criticism.

Kapha is structure and provides lubrication. In balance it evokes feelings of love, calm and forgiveness. When out of balance it evokes feelings of greed, attachment, lust and envy.

No matter what your predominant constitution is, all newly-birthed mothers have to deal with an imbalance of postpartum vata. In order to regain balance after birth, it is essential to counteract these innate qualities of vata through a healing diet, ample rest, oil massage, herbs and a meditative environment.

The 20 Physical Qualities of Creation

According to Ayurveda, there are 20 physical qualities of creation. These 20 qualities, or *gunas*, are broken down into 10 opposing pairs that function together. Our world is made up of these opposing forces, their constant play has a central role in shaping our experience in the physical world. Without the opposing forces of male and female, day and night, how would this beautiful creation even exist?

The fundamental qualities of creation are the foundation in which we can learn to balance our health. None of these qualities are better than the other, all have their rightful place in creation. When trying to regain balance over a specific quality, you need to apply the opposite quality to the situation. For example, if you are feeling really cold, you need to find warmth. You can do this by putting on a heavy jacket, drinking warm tea, sitting by a fireplace, or a combination of all three! This same principal of invoking the opposite quality applies to all 10 antagonistic pairs.

The qualities that result from giving birth are light, sharp, cold, dense, dry, rough, hard, mobile, subtle and clear. In order to have a strong postpartum recovery, we need to focus on using their opposites in order to bring your health back into balance. We can do this though an informed postpartum diet, massage, and herbs, as well as resting and nesting.

The 10 qualities on the left side are imbalanced through the act of birthing and breastfeeding. You can regain your balanced health by counteracting them with their opposing qualities, which are shown on the right side.

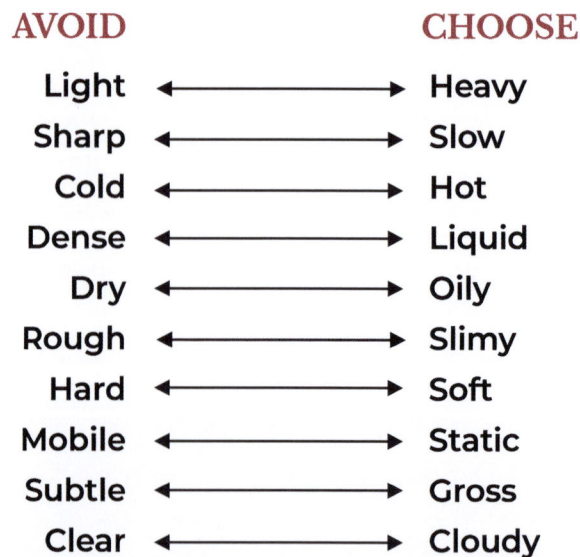

AVOID		CHOOSE
Light	←→	Heavy
Sharp	←→	Slow
Cold	←→	Hot
Dense	←→	Liquid
Dry	←→	Oily
Rough	←→	Slimy
Hard	←→	Soft
Mobile	←→	Static
Subtle	←→	Gross
Clear	←→	Cloudy

The 3 Subtle Qualities of Creation

There are 3 subtle qualities that are manifest in all forms of creation, *sattva*, *rajas* and *tamas*. These 3 subtle qualities have a powerful effect on the mind and life force.

Sattva is the harmonizing force of creation. It is the quality of healing, light, life and love, and the spiritual force that allows our consciousness to evolve. This quality imparts virtues of faith, honesty, self-control, clarity and purity.

Rajas is the active force that stimulates change. It is the quality of passion, agitation and transition. *Rajas* is dynamic movement, and lacks stability and consistency. This quality gives rise to the emotional fluctuations of attraction and repulsion, love and hate, fear and desire.

Tamas is the passive force of inertia that sustains previous activity. It is the quality of darkness, non-feeling and death, the lower force that drags us down into ignorance and attachment. This quality causes dullness, degradation, heaviness and stagnation.

These 3 qualities are intertwined in creation and tend to hold their natures for a period of time, such as in the cycle of the day (sattva), twilight (rajas) and night (tamas).

Cultivating a Sattvic Lifestyle After Birth

Healing naturally arises when you are in a sattvic state. Cultivating a sattvic lifestyle for at least the first 6 weeks postpartum will help you maintain balance in your body and mind, avoid mental/emotional disturbances, digestive issues, and overall help your postpartum healing experience.

You can achieve this by:
- Eating postpartum appropriate meals
- Getting enough rest
- Daily oil massage
- Yoga Nidra (yogic sleep meditation)

- Pranayama (breathing exercises)
- Listening to relaxing music
- Staying away from television and violent movies
- Maintaining a meditative atmosphere

By maintaining a sattvic lifestyle during your postpartum recovery, you will regain balance, therefore allowing your body to rejuvenate to its fullest potential.

Chapter 2
The Ayurvedic Postpartum Diet

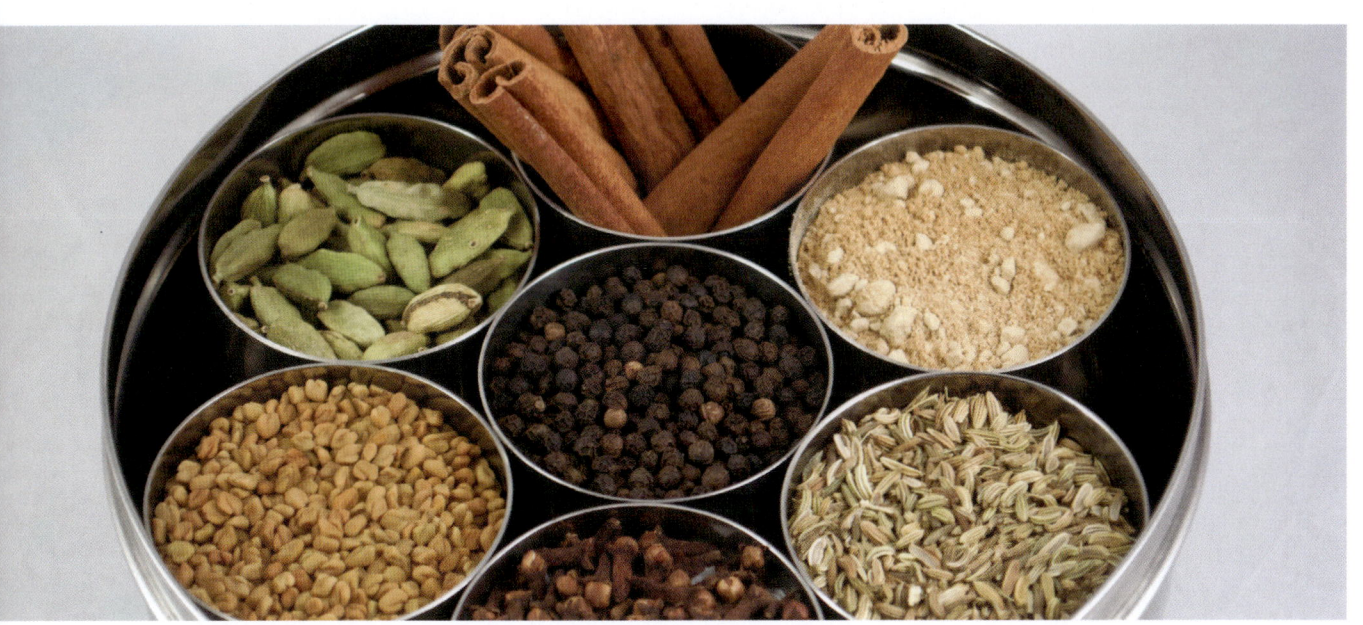

Eating a nourishing, digestible postpartum diet is the single most important facet of your postpartum recovery. The quality of your diet after birth will have a significant impact on your postnatal health as well as your breast milk supply.

Within this chapter, you will learn how to cook and eat the best diet for strong postnatal rejuvenation. Included are the 4 phases of the Ayurvedic postpartum diet, Ayurvedic diet energetics, best and worst foods for postpartum, the best foods for vitality, and how to transition back to a regular diet. By learning these underlying principles, you will have a greater understanding of *why* Ayurvedic postnatal recipes are so healing after birth.

Ayurvedic Diet Energetics

Every food has its own unique attributes that will affect its taste as well as its action on the body. The concepts of taste (*rasa*), energy (*virya*) and latent, post-digestive effect (*vipak*) are all important concepts to understand in order to use diet as a vehicle for self-healing.

Taste (rasa)

Taste, or *rasa*, is experienced by the tongue directly after putting something in the mouth. Rasa is the first step in the digestive process.

There are 6 tastes inherent in all food: sweet, sour, salty, bitter, pungent and astringent. The first three: sweet, sour and salty are upbuilding in nature and therefore beneficial for postpartum rejuvenation. The last three: bitter, pungent and astringent are cleansing in nature and therefore not conducive to postpartum rejuvenation. Although it is still important to incorporate all 6 tastes to have a balanced meal, during postpartum recovery, we lean heavily on the rebuilding tastes of **sweet**, **sour** and **salty**.

Energy (virya)

When any food, herb, or spice is put in the mouth, we first experience its taste. Next we experience its heating or cooling energy *(virya)*. Sometimes this happens immediately in the mouth, like cayenne or peppermint. More often, however, virya happens in the stomach. Sweet, astringent and bitter tastes have a cooling energy, while salty, sour and pungent (spicy) tastes have a heating energy.

In Ayurvedic cooking, we consider the heating and cooling effects of every element of our meal to create the perfect balance for healing. When in postpartum recovery, the focus is on maintaining a **heating** action on the body, which naturally becomes cold from the birth.

Latent Effect (vipak)

Vipak is the latent post-digestive effect of taste on the body, mind, and consciousness. It is the final energy that is produced from the food that is consumed. Sweet and salty tastes have a sweet vipak. Sour taste has a sour vipak. Pungent, astringent and bitter tastes all have pungent post-digestive effects.

By understanding your food's taste, heating or cooling energy, and its post-digestive effect, you will be empowered to make good decisions about what foods will bring you into balance and which are best avoided to maintain your health.

Cultivating Strong Digestion After Birth

Cultivating strong digestion after birth, is of central importance in maintaining a balanced state of health. The concept of digestive fire, or *agni*, has both a physical, as well as subtle nature. Agni is the transformative energy that assimilates that which is "not self" into "self."

Agni is responsible for digesting not only your food, but also your experiences. When agni is strong, you efficiently assimilate all the nutrients in your food, leading to vibrant health. Similarly, with a strong digestive fire, you are able to process your experiences with clarity, leading to a balanced mental state.

Conversely, when your digestive power is weak, your body is not able to fully digest the food you eat. This leads to a build up of toxins in the body and mind. When toxins are present, the mind can become dull and cloudy and the body's digestive process can become clogged. This leads to gas, bloating and unhealthy elimination patterns that can lead to emotional imbalances as well.

Follow these rules for proper digestion:

- Allow time between meals to properly digest. 3 hours for most foods, 30-45 minutes for fruit.
- Don't drink too much liquid with your meal. It's like throwing water on a fire, and will dampen you digestive fire. Especially if it is cold!
- Drinking warm fluids is especially important during postpartum, room temperature should be the absolute coldest!
- Don't use ice.
- Avoid carbonated beverages. These *air* bubbles will surely contribute to the imbalance of air (vata) that you are already dealing with.
- Practice mindful eating: chew your food well, and avoid TV etc. while eating, as well as walking and even talking.

After birth, your body's internal fire will be diminished for some time. The energy it takes to birth a human being into this world is immense. Your digestion will need some encouragement to be rekindled gracefully, and regain its strength after such an amazing feat!

Most people in our society today are unaware of the influence our digestive capacity has on our postpartum recovery. By not understanding this fact, we see many imbalances with postnatal mothers and newborns that have unfortunately become commonplace. Many health problems new mothers face can be easily avoided by having a strong digestive fire and eating a supportive postpartum diet. Without these fundamentals in place, it will be challenging to regain vitality after birth.

Food Combining

An important element to maintaining a healthy digestive fire, is understanding proper food combining. Not all foods work together synergistically. Some foods digest quickly, while others take more time. If you combine foods that have different digestive processes, it can dampen the digestive fire and create unwanted toxins in your system. For example, you should never eat fruit with your meal. Fruit has a fast digestive process, while vegetables, proteins and grains take much longer to digest. Combining these foods will create fermentation in the stomach, which leads to gas, bloating, toxic build-up and poor digestion.

It's important to understand which foods combine well together in order to maintain a healthy digestive environment. Outlined below are the food combining rules that need to be followed to ensure the proper assimilation of your food's nutrients.

- Eat fruit by itself.
- Eat melon by itself (don't combine with other types of fruit).
- Don't combine different forms of dairy, like cheese and milk.
- Milk is a complete food and is best taken by itself. It can be combined with sweet grains and tapioca. Avoid mixing milk with salt.

- Avoid mixing eggs with dairy, meat and fruit.
- Avoid mixing citrus with dairy. It curdles!
- Don't cook honey, it will become toxic.
- Don't mix starch with dairy, eggs, fruit, or dates.

Cultivating Vitality Through Proper Diet

Within our body we carry a very deep and subtle form of vitality. This vital essence is known in Ayurveda as *ojas*. Ojas is like our body's natural honey: it is the purest essence resulting from the nourishment we take into our system. It is also directly related to our immunity. Having strong ojas also means having strong resistance to infection and disease. This subtle form of vitality acts as a protective shield and helps ward off stress, as well as imbalances of both the body and the mind.

It is important to be mindful of your ojas after birth. As It can easily become depleted through stress, excessive activity, weak digestion and bad dietary choices. In order to protect your most subtle essence of vitality, you need to be mindful and give yourself proper rest, self-care and nourishment. Postpartum recovery, above all, is a process of rebuilding that supply of vital energy.

The most important element of building your ojas through diet is cultivating a strong digestive fire. There are also some foods that are especially suited for increasing vitality, provided you introduce them to your system in the right way.

The most notable foods for increasing your postnatal vitality include:
- Ghee
- Dates
- Almonds
- Cashews
- Raw Cow's Milk
- Saffron

There is an abundance of recipes crafted to specifically rebuild your vitality in this cookbook. As long as you follow proper digestive guidelines, as well as the recipes in Mama's Menu, you should be good to go!

Healing Postpartum Foods

Each food has its own intrinsic characteristics. Circling back around to our Ayurvedic basics, each food will have specific physical qualities such as heavy or light, dry or moist, hot or cold etc. Their taste could be sweet or sour, bitter or pungent, salty or astringent. They could have a heating or cooling effect on the body, and they could best balance vata, pitta, or kapha.

Taking all of these things into consideration, and favoring the characteristics best suited to postnatal rejuvenation, we come to our healing postpartum foods list.

Seasonings
- Basil
- Cumin
- Clove
- Citrus peel
- Cardamom
- Cinnamon
- Fennel
- Fenugreek
- Licorice
- Garlic (browned in oil)
- Ginger
- Marjoram
- Allspice
- Nutmeg
- Black pepper
- Paprika
- Dill
- Tamarind
- Tarragon
- Turmeric
- Ajwain
- Asafoetida (Hing)
- Saffron
- Vanilla beans
- Cayenne

Fats
- Ghee
- Butter
- Sesame oil
- Olive oil
- Coconut milk

Fruits
- Sweet fresh fruits & juices
- Dates
- Avocado
- Coconut
- Lemon
- Lime

Proteins
- Boiled milk
- Unfermented cheeses (cottage, ricotta, fresh paneer)
- Sesame seeds
- Almonds
- Split mung beans
- Urad dal
- Soaked & pureed beans
- Garbanzo flour
- Quinoa
- Amaranth

Vegetables
- Asparagus
- Root vegetables
- Summer squash
- Winter squash
- Artichoke
- Cilantro
- Okra
- Fennel bulb
- Fenugreek leaves
- Dark leafy greens

Carbs
- Basmati rice
- Unleavened Wheat
- Tapioca
- Oats
- Yams
- Sweet potatoes

Sweeteners
- Molasses
- Raw cane sugar
- Coconut sugar
- Maple syrup
- Jaggery

Foods to Avoid After Birth

Just as there are foods that promote postpartum healing, there are also foods that can obstruct the postnatal healing process. Below is the list of foods to avoid for *at least* 6 weeks after birth.

- Raw foods
- Dry foods
- Cruciferous vegetables (brassicas)
- Nightshades
- Fermented foods
- Leavening agents
- Chocolate
- Caffeine
- Carbonated beverages
- Mushrooms
- Leftovers
- Cold foods
- Frozen foods
- Meat
- Alcohol

When you do decide to add some of these foods back into your diet, remember to observe how both you and your baby (if breastfeeding) feel. If you feel gassy or your baby seems uncomfortable, you may need to wait longer than just 6 weeks after birth before expanding your menu options. The best thing to do is introduce one new food at a time and be mindful of the effects it has on you and your baby.

The 4 Phases of an Ayurvedic Postpartum Diet

Postpartum rejuvenation is broken down into 4 distinct phases. This is needed to nurture the flame of your digestion into a healthy fire that can easily transform nutrients into vitality.

Days 1-3: Cleansing & Digestion

For the first 3 days after birth, your body is focusing on cleansing. Your milk hasn't yet come in, and your body is focused on flushing out your uterus from the birth. Now is the time to use extra turmeric and some pungent spices to support cleansing and stoking the digestive fire. Your food should be very well cooked, with lots of ghee and digestive spices. Focus mainly on porridges, puddings, thin soups and hot teas. It is better to limit vegetables for the first few days because of their inherent astringency.

Days 4-10: Digestion & Lactation

Once your milk comes in, the focus shifts away from cleansing, and moves into cultivating digestion and building your milk supply. Tone down the use of turmeric, as it is cleansing in nature. Continue to eat an abundance of ghee and digestive spices in your meals. The focus is still on soupy foods. Vegetables can be introduced with caution. Creamy drinks and desserts with adequate spices can be enjoyed as well.

Days 11-21: Lactation & Rejuvenation

By this point in your postpartum recovery, your digestive fire should have strength. While still supporting digestion, the focus now shifts toward lactation and rejuvenation. Vegetables are welcome at this stage, as well as fresh, unfermented cheese, soaked nuts and unleavened flatbreads.

Days 22-42: Rejuvenation

The final phase of your postpartum recovery is solely focused on rebuilding your health. By this phase you should have strong digestion and a great breast milk supply. Now is the time to focus on making sure you are eating to rebuild your strength and vitality. More complex homemade foods can now be enjoyed, such as pasta, whole beans, creamy vegetable stir-fries, and hummus.

Transitioning Back to a Regular Diet

After your 4th trimester is complete, it is important to gradually transition back to a regular diet. By slowly re-introducing more complex foods, you give your digestive fire time to build its strength and ability to handle the complex foods you have been patiently avoiding. If you just go back to eating pizza and ice cream right away, it's likely your digestion and breast milk will be compromised.

In order to maintain a strong digestive fire when transitioning back to a regular diet, you need to stick with your digestive protocol. Drink some digestive tea, remember your food combining rules, and make sure you are allowing time in between meals for complete digestion.

The best way to successfully transition back to a regular diet, is by introducing one new food a day and observe how your body responds to it. That way you can be sure what it was that gave you, or your breastfed baby, trouble. If you experience gas, bloating or elimination problems, back off of whatever food you have introduced, as your body may not be ready for it yet.

If you are breastfeeding, you may find that certain foods may not agree with your baby, even after your 6 week postpartum recovery is over. This is totally normal. You may even need to avoid certain foods for the entire time you breastfeed. By watching your diet closely, you will learn what foods, if any, you may need to continue avoiding for the time being. This conscious practice of observing dietary changes and effects will serve you and your little one well into the future.

Rebalancing After Birth

Through understanding the aforementioned concepts, we are ready to sum up how to best rebalance after birth.

The two elements that are significantly increased by the birthing process are air and space, the two elements that make up the vata dosha. Because of this, we need an excess of fire, water and earth to rebalance after birth.

The physical qualities of vata are light, subtle, dry, rough, mobile, cold, and irregular. All of these qualities are strongly accentuated after birth and need their opposites to bring them back into harmony.

In order to counteract dryness, new mothers need an abundance of healthy oils, both inside and out. To balance roughness, you need soft, easy to digest foods. To combat the mobile quality of vata, lots of rest is needed. To prevent coldness from settling into your system, make sure everything in your internal and external environment is warm. This includes foods, liquids, hot baths as well as the air. To impede irregularity, a daily routine will bring much needed rhythm to your life. By applying vata's opposites in this way, you as a new mother, can find your balance once again.

It is best to focus on foods and experiences that are regenerative in nature and carry a high (sattvic) vibration. This is important while you are rebuilding your body after birth. This is why an Ayurvedic postpartum diet is vegetarian. Meat, as well as fermented foods, processed foods and leftovers, all have a degenerative (tamasic) quality. Degenerative foods and environments are best avoided during postpartum rejuvenation.

A proper diet is crucial for a healthy postpartum recovery. In order to do this you need:

1. A strong digestive fire to completely process your foods and experiences. You can do this through eating well-cooked, warm, soupy foods with lots of digestive spices and oils.
2. Get to know what foods and spices are best suited for your postpartum healing. Focus on foods with sweet, sour, and salty tastes. Also, make sure to keep your food and environment warm, not cold. This will pacify the unsettled vata dosha and bring balance to your system once again.
3. Eat foods that specifically build your vitality (ojas). This is your chance to hit the reset button on your physical health. In order for you to both nourish yourself as well as your baby, you need to eat nutrient dense foods that you can digest easily.

Once you regain your digestive strength, you can rebuild your body's vitality, as well as your breast milk supply. Your vitality is the cornerstone of your baby's well-being. The energy you put into your postpartum healing will undoubtedly benefit your baby as well.

Chapter 3

Getting Prepared

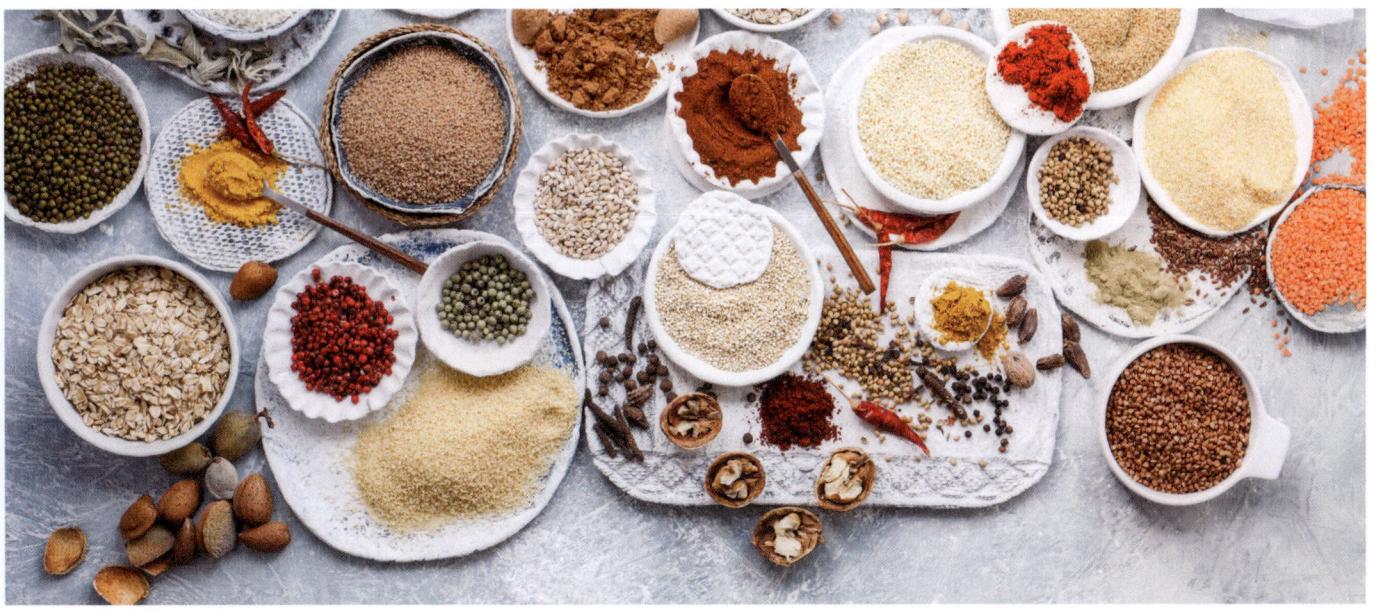

In order to maximize your postpartum recovery, you need to make sure you have your postpartum diet plan in place before the baby arrives. If you do not plan in advance, you will most likely put yourself in a serious disadvantage. Once your baby is born, it's almost impossible to organize and plan anything!

If you would like to get the most benefit from your healing postnatal diet, it is best to have gathered all necessary ingredients and equipment beforehand, as well as having a diet plan in place. It is also important to consider who will be cooking, especially for the first few weeks after delivery.

Kitchen Tools

There are certain cooking tools that will prove their worth when utilizing this cookbook. For example, If you don't have a lot of cooking support available after the birth, a programmable slow-cooker is essential to manage your nourishment. Even if you do have ample support, programmable cookers can make life A LOT easier!

Below is a list of cooking equipment needed to easily make the recipes in this cookbook.

- VitaClay programmable cooker. This "slow" cooker cooks twice as fast as a regular crockpot and is made out of unglazed clay, enabling you to extract extra nutrients while increasing digestibility.
- High quality blender (Vitamix)
- Electric spice/coffee grinder - dedicated for grinding spices
- 1 large cast-iron frying pan
- 1 small and 2 medium saucepans with lids
- 1 large soup pot with lid
- 1 small and 1 medium frying pan
- 1 medium to large ceramic non-stick pot and medium skillet (Green Pan)
- Wooden spoon and spatula
- Metal spatula
- Rubber spatula
- Measuring cups and spoons
- Mixing bowls
- Loaf pan
- 8"X8" baking pan
- Cookie sheet
- Sharp knives
- Cutting board
- Cheese cloth or thin muslin cloth for straining
- Small and medium strainer
- Hand held electric mixer

Mama's Menu Grocery List

I encourage you to browse through this cookbook, pick out the recipes you know you want to eat and make a shopping list accordingly. Below is a complete shopping list, with all the ingredients represented in Mama's Menu.

Herbs and Spices
- Fennel seed
- Cumin seed and powder
- Fenugreek seed and powder
- Cayenne powder
- Cardamom pods and powder
- Fresh ginger root and ginger powder
- Nutmeg powder
- Whole cloves and powder
- Allspice powder
- Asafoetida powder (hing)
- Garlic cloves
- Black peppercorns and black pepper powder
- Fresh and dried basil
- Saffron
- Turmeric powder
- Coriander powder
- Cinnamon sticks and powder
- Ajwain seeds
- Tarragon
- Salt
- Coconut aminos
- Fresh mint
- Vanilla powder and/or vanilla extract
- Rooibos (red tea)
- Tamarind paste
- Crystalized ginger
- Curry powder
- Black mustard seed
- Garam masala

Nuts and Seeds
- Shredded coconut and coconut milk
- Whole raw almonds and blanched almond flour
- Pecans
- Cashews
- Hulled, white sesame seeds
- Tahini

Oils
- Ghee
- Unsalted butter
- Unrefined sesame oil

Grains
- Basmati rice
- Cream of rice
- Quinoa
- Garbanzo bean flour
- Tapioca
- Cream of wheat (farina)
- Rolled oats
- Amaranth
- Whole wheat pastry flour
- Semolina or quinoa pasta
- Barley
- Rice noodles
- Arrowroot starch
- Rice flour
- Oat flour

- Yellow split peeled mung dal
- Green whole mung beans
- Channa dal
- Black beans
- Toor dal
- Urad dal
- Tofu
- Great Northern Beans

Fruits
- Apples (cooked only!)
- Pears (cooked only!)
- Dates
- Strawberries
- Banana
- Fig jam
- Dried apricots
- Raisins
- Avocado
- Lemon juice
- Lime juice

Sweeteners
- Coconut sugar
- Jaggery
- Maple syrup
- Turbinado cane sugar
- Molasses
- Honey

Vegetables
- Cilantro
- Butternut squash
- Fennel bulb
- Carrots
- Beets
- Sweet potatoes
- Yams
- Spinach
- Swiss chard
- Pumpkin
- Sugar snap peas
- Mung sprouts
- Zucchini

Dairy
- Cream-top milk
- Yogurt
- Goat chèvre
- Heavy whipping cream

TIP: It is better to buy spices in bulk, whenever possible. Spices can be pricey, and you will use a lot of them in your postpartum diet! Not only will buying in bulk be cheaper, it will save on packaging as well.

Where to Find Unfamiliar Ingredients

If you are unfamiliar with Indian cooking, some of the ingredients may be foreign to you. Below is a list of less-common ingredients and where you might find them in your locality. All of these ingredients you can buy online.

1. Yellow Mung Dal (split and peeled mung beans) - sometimes found in health food stores. Otherwise, Indian grocers and Asian markets.

2. Urad Dal (split and peeled urad beans) - available at Indian grocers and Asian markets.

3. Chana Dal (split garbanzo beans) - sometimes found at your local health food store, otherwise Indian grocers and Asian markets.

4. Toor Dal (split pigeon peas) - found at Indian grocers and Asian markets.

5. Jaggery -This iron-rich, buttery raw sugar is only found at Indian grocers and sometimes, Asian markets.

6. Ghee - can be found in health food stores and Indian grocers.

7. Coconut Sugar - unprocessed raw sugar which can be found at your local health food store.

8. Vanilla powder - found at your local health food store.

9. Saffron - can be found in health food stores and Indian grocers.

10. Turmeric -can be found in health food stores, Asian and Indian markets.

11. Cardamom - can be found in some health food stores, as well as Indian grocers.

12. Hing (Asafoetida) - this unique smelling Indian spice is commonly used as a replacement for onions and garlic. It can sometimes be found in health food stores, but is readily available at Indian grocers.

13. Crystalized Ginger - available at health food stores.

14. Garam Masala - available at some health food stores, as well as Indian grocers.

15. Tamarind Paste - available at some health food stores, as well as Indian grocers, and Asian markets.

16. Coconut Aminos - available at health food stores.

17. Garbanzo Bean Flour -available at health food stores and Indian grocers.

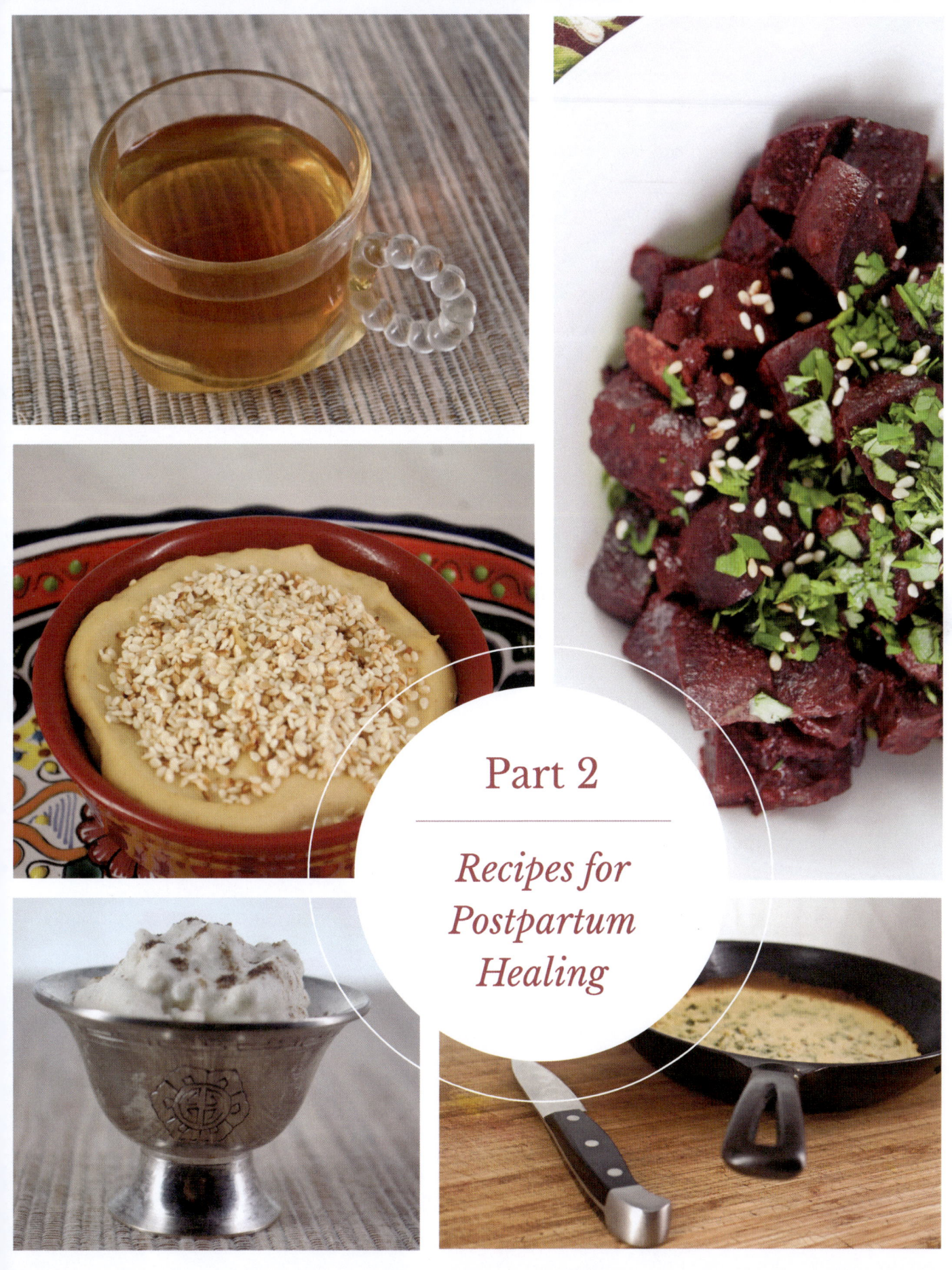

Part 2

Recipes for Postpartum Healing

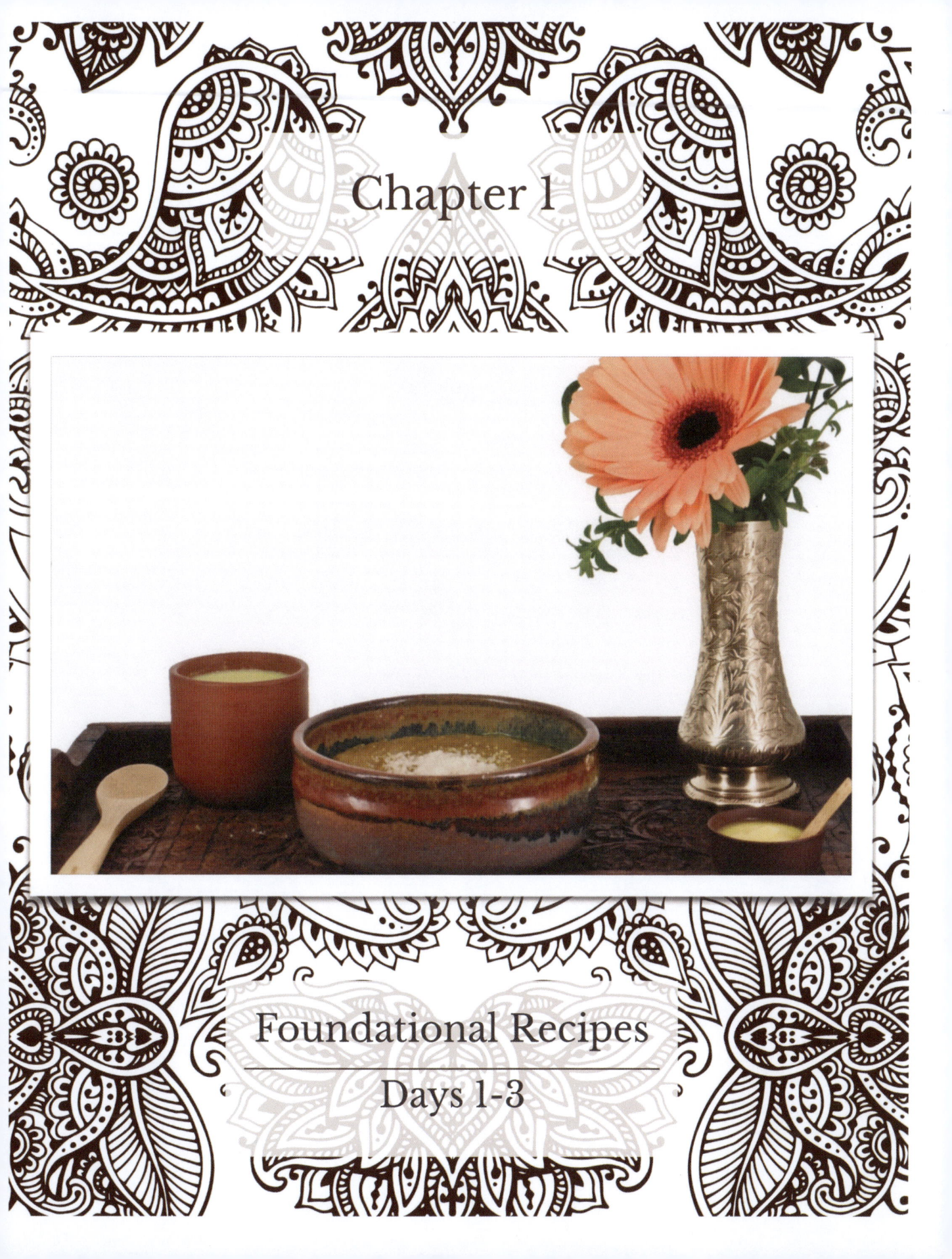

Chapter 1

Foundational Recipes

Days 1-3

Strong Fenugreek Tea

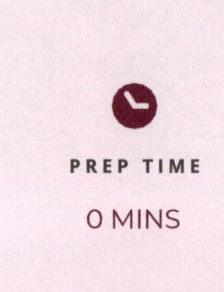

PREP TIME
0 MINS

COOK TIME
10 MINS

SERVES
2

INGREDIENTS

4 cups water
1 tablespoon fenugreek seeds
2 teaspoons maple syrup

INSTRUCTIONS

1. Bring water and fenugreek seeds to a boil.
2. Reduce heat and simmer for 10 minutes.
3. Strain and stir in maple syrup.
4. Serve hot for the first few days after birth.

First Days Rice Congee

PREP TIME
5 MINS

COOK TIME
6 HOURS

SERVES
2-3

INGREDIENTS

8 cups water
1 cup basmati rice
1 1/2 cups coconut sugar or jaggery
1/2 cup ghee or unsalted butter*
2 teaspoons ginger powder
1 teaspoon cinnamon powder
3/4 teaspoon cardamom powder
1/2 teaspoon clove powder
1/2 teaspoon black pepper
1/2 teaspoon turmeric powder
pinch of cayenne (optional)

* Use sesame oil if vegan

INSTRUCTIONS

1. Rinse rice several times under warm running water until clear. Drain.
2. Add all ingredients to a your VitaClay cooker. Stew for 4+ hours. For a regular crockpot cook for 6-8 hours.
3. When the consistency is gelatinous, your porridge is ready! Take off heat and serve hot.

Note: This recipe ideally will be started at the onset of labor. If you plan to cook it on the stovetop, it will need to cook for several hours to achieve the gelatinous consistency. Add additional water if necessary.

Mother's Milk

PREP TIME
0 MINS

COOK TIME
20 MINS

SERVES
4

INGREDIENTS

8 cups cream top milk (non-homogenized)
1 tablespoon whole cloves
1 teaspoon black pepper
2 tablespoons cardamom pods
1/2 teaspoon turmeric powder
1 tablespoon ginger powder
1 teaspoon fennel seed
1 tablespoon turbinado sugar
1 tablespoon ghee

INSTRUCTIONS

1. Add milk to a heavy bottomed saucepan (ceramic non-stick is ideal).
2. Bring to a boil, watching carefully for it to not boil over.
3. Turn heat to low and add the remaining ingredients.
4. Simmer partially covered for 20 minutes.
5. Strain and serve first thing in the morning or before bed.
6. Refrigerate for up to 3 days. Always serve hot.

Vital Garlic Chutney

PREP TIME
2 MINS

COOK TIME
7 MINS

SERVES
16

INGREDIENTS

1/2 cup garlic cloves (peeled)
3 tablespoons ghee
1 cup shredded coconut
4 tablespoons black pepper (ground)
1 teaspoon coriander powder
1 teaspoon salt
1/2 tablespoon lemon juice

INSTRUCTIONS

1. Melt ghee in small frying pan over medium heat. Add garlic.
2. Turn heat down to medium-low and slowly brown garlic. Stir from time to time to ensure all sides for each clove are browned evenly.
3. Add all ingredients to food processor and process until a uniform consistency is achieved.
4. Eat liberally with meals directly after birth.

Raab

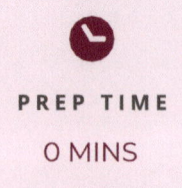

PREP TIME 0 MINS

COOK TIME 10 MINS

SERVES 2-3

INGREDIENTS

4 cups water
3 tablespoons coconut sugar
1/4 cup wheat farina
3 tablespoons ghee
1/2 teaspoon ginger powder
1/8 teaspoon nutmeg
3 tablespoons almond flour (blanched)

INSTRUCTIONS

1. Heat water and sugar together in a small saucepan until well combined.
2. In a medium-sized saucepan, melt ghee and add farina and spices. Cook on medium-low heat for three minutes, stirring regularly.
3. Take pan off heat and add the water-sugar mixture, stirring constantly with a whisk.
4. Return saucepan to medium-low heat, and cook for another 3-5 minutes, or until slightly thickened.
5. Stir in almond flour and serve.

Cream of Rice Cereal with Dates

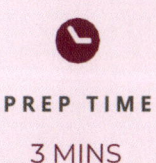

PREP TIME
3 MINS

COOK TIME
30+ MINS

SERVES
2

INGREDIENTS

1/2 cup cream of rice
3 cups water
1 tablespoon ghee
1/3 teaspoon cinnamon
1/4 teaspoon ginger powder
1/4 teaspoon nutmeg powder
1/4 teaspoon clove powder
3 dates (pitted and chopped)
2 tablespoons coconut sugar

INSTRUCTIONS

1. Bring cream of rice and water to a boil. Stir periodically to avoid clumping and sticking.
2. Turn heat down to medium low. Stir in spices and sugar. Cover.
3. Cook for 30-45 minutes, or until throughly cooked.
4. Turn off heat and add chopped dates.
5. Serve hot

Note: This recipe is great for a programable VitaClay. Program the night before and have it ready when you wake up in the morning!

Healing Mung Dal Soup

PREP TIME
35 MINS

COOK TIME
45+ MINS

SERVES
2

INGREDIENTS

1/4 cup yellow mung dal
4 cups water
3 tablespoons ghee
1/4 teaspoon turmeric
2 garlic cloves (minced)
1 teaspoon fresh ginger (grated)
1 teaspoon cumin powder
3/4 teaspoon fenugreek powder
1/2 teaspoon clove powder
1 teaspoon coconut sugar
2 pinches cayenne
3/4 teaspoon salt
1/2 teaspoon lemon juice

INSTRUCTIONS

1. Rinse mung dal under warm running water until clear.
2. Soak mung dal for 30 minutes. Drain.
3. Add dal, water, turmeric and 1 tablespoon of ghee to heavy bottomed saucepan.
4. Bring to a boil and turn down to a simmer. Partially cover and cook for 45 minutes to 1 hour. Alternately, cook 20 minutes in a pressure cooker or 2 hours in your VitaClay.
5. Add the rest of the ghee to a small frying pan on medium heat. Add garlic and turn down to medium low to slowly brown.
6. Once garlic has begun to turn color, add grated ginger, cumin, fenugreek and clove. Stir until fragrant.
7. Add sugar and cayenne and stir. Once the sugar caramelizes to a reddish brown, add entire contents into the soup.
8. Add salt and lemon juice. Stir until well combined and let sit for 5 minutes for the flavors to infuse into the soup.
9. Serve hot.

Calming Kitchari

PREP TIME
10 MINS

COOK TIME
1+ HOUR

SERVES
2-3

INGREDIENTS

1/4 cup yellow mung dal
3/4 cup basmati rice
5 cups water
3 tablespoons ghee or sesame oil
1/2 teaspoon turmeric

Spice Mixture:
1 garlic clove (minced)
1/2 teaspoon black pepper
1/4 teaspoon fenugreek powder
1 1/2 teaspoons cumin powder
1/8 teaspoon clove powder
1/8 teaspoon ajwain
1/2 teaspoon of *Mama's Masala (pg 46)* or garam masala
3 tablespoons cilantro (chopped)
1 1/2 tablespoons shredded coconut
1/4 cup water

INSTRUCTIONS

1. Rinse rice and mung dal under warm running water until clear. Drain.
2. Add rice, dal, water, turmeric and 1 tablespoon of ghee to a medium saucepan or slow cooker.
3. Cook until very soft and mushy. On the stovetop, for about an hour, 2 hours in your VitaClay cooker.

For the spice mixture:

4. Add cilantro, coconut and 1/4 cup of water to a blender and blend well.
5. Heat remaining ghee in small frying pan on medium heat.
6. Add minced garlic and fry until lightly browned.
7. Add cumin, fenugreek, ajwain, and masala and stir until fragrant.
8. Pour in cilantro-coconut mixture. Add clove powder and black pepper. Allow to simmer for 30 seconds.
9. Pour the spice mixture into the pot of kitchari. Add salt and stir until very well until combined.
10. Allow the flavors to mingle for 5 minutes.
11. Serve warm.

Almond Kheer

PREP TIME
6 + HOURS

COOK TIME
5 MINS

SERVES
2

INGREDIENTS

2 tablespoons almonds or almond flour (blanched)
2 cups milk
1 pinch saffron
4 tablespoons turbinado sugar
2 teaspoons ghee
1/4 teaspoon cardamom powder

INSTRUCTIONS

1. Soak almonds overnight and peel (As a shortcut you can use blanched almond flour).
2. Soak saffron for 10 minutes in a tablespoon of milk.
3. Blend 1/2 cup of milk with almonds or almond flour.
4. In a small non-stick or heavy bottomed saucepan, add milk and almond mixture and bring to a boil.
5. Turn down heat to medium-low and add ghee, sugar, saffron mixture and cardamom.
6. Cook 5 minutes. Serve hot.

Crustless Apple Pie

PREP TIME
10 MINS

COOK TIME
20 MINS

SERVES
2-3

INGREDIENTS

6 apples
2 cups water
3 tablespoons coconut sugar or jaggery
1/2 teaspoon clove powder
1 teaspoon cinnamon powder
2 tablespoons ghee

Crumble Mix
2 tablespoons almond flour
1 tablespoon coconut sugar
1/8 teaspoon cinnamon
Pinch of nutmeg

INSTRUCTIONS

1. Wash, peel, core and chop apples into bite size pieces.
2. Add water, chopped apples, sugar, ghee and spices to a saucepan and bring to a boil.
3. Turn down to a simmer and cook with the lid off until apples are soft and the liquid has thickened, about 20 minutes.
4. Turn off stove and stir in the crumble mix until well combined.
5. Serve warm for breakfast or as a snack.

Mama's Masala

PREP TIME
20 MINS

COOK TIME
15 MINS

SERVES
30

INGREDIENTS

3 tablespoons shredded coconut
4 tablespoons sesame seeds
2 teaspoons cumin powder
1/2 teaspoon coriander powder
1 teaspoon fennel seed
1/4 teaspoon saffron threads
1 teaspoon cinnamon powder
3/4 teaspoon clove powder
1 teaspoon cardamom powder
3/4 teaspoon ground black pepper
1/2 teaspoon ginger powder

INSTRUCTIONS

1. Dry roast the sesame seeds until golden brown. Repeat with the coconut.
2. Dry roast cumin, coriander, and fennel together until a few shades darker.
3. Grind coconut, sesame, cumin, coriander, and fennel to a powder using spice grinder or mortar and pestle.
4. Mix in remaining ingredients.
5. Store in an airtight jar.

Note: Add to any recipe calling for garam masala. Additionally you can sprinkle 1 teaspoon over any meal to add flavor and digestibility.

Ghee

PREP TIME 5 MINS

COOK TIME 15 MINS

SERVES 20+

INGREDIENTS

1 lb. unsalted butter

INSTRUCTIONS

1. Put the butter in a medium sized saucepan on medium heat until the butter melts.
2. Once the butter begins to boil rapidly, turn down heat until you have a softer boil. The butter will foam and sputter for a few minutes but then will start to quiet down.
3. In 12-15 minutes, it will begin to smell like popcorn and turn a clear golden color. When the ghee is finished, you will be able to see the bottom of the pot very clearly.
4. Once you have clear golden liquid, take the pot off the heat, as it can burn very easily at this stage.
5. Let ghee cool until just warm.
6. Skim any foam off the top and save if you desire. This foam has medicinal qualities and can be eaten on rice.
7. Pour ghee through a thin cotton cloth, handkerchief or a few layers of cheesecloth into a glass container.
8. Cover with a tight lid. Ghee does not need refrigeration.

Chapter 2

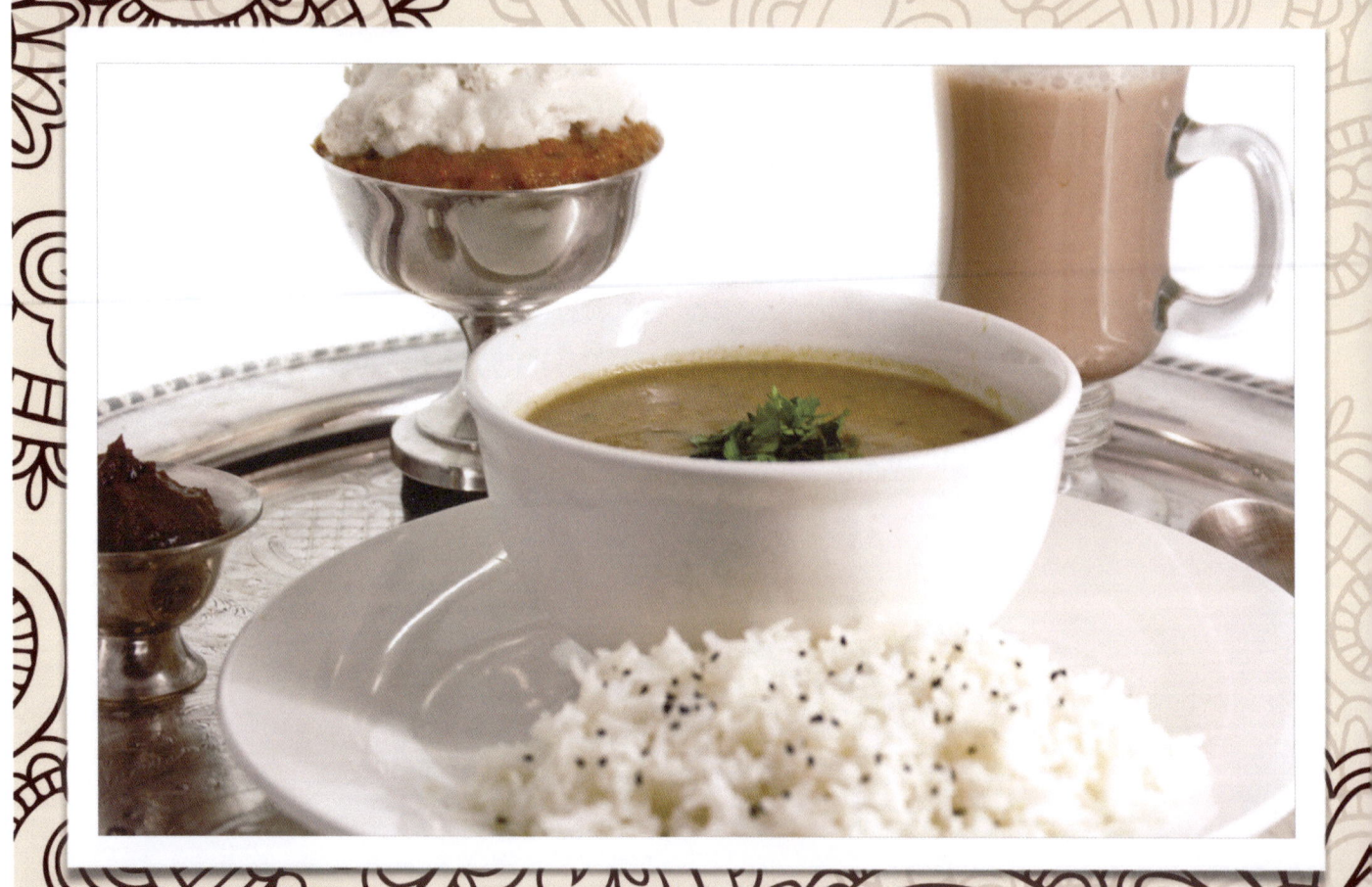

Digestion & Lactation
Days 4-10

Simple Lactation Tea

PREP TIME
0 MINS

COOK TIME
5 MINS

SERVES
8

INGREDIENTS

2/3 teaspoon fennel seeds
1/3 teaspoon fenugreek seeds
8 cups water

INSTRUCTIONS

1. Boil water.
2. Add fennel and fenugreek to water and let steep for 10 minutes.
3. Strain and pour into an insulated mug to drink throughout the day.

Mother's Red Chai

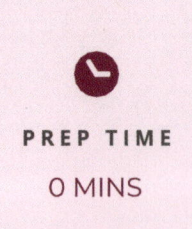

PREP TIME
0 MINS

COOK TIME
7 MINS

SERVES
2

INGREDIENTS

1" piece of fresh ginger (grated)
2 tablespoons cardamom pods
1 teaspoon clove buds
2" stick cinnamon
1/4 teaspoon black pepper
1/4 teaspoon fennel seeds
1 cup cream-top milk*
1 cup water
1 tablespoon rooibos tea

*Substitute almond milk if vegan

INSTRUCTIONS

1. Bring milk and water to a boil and add spices. Turn down to a simmer and cover.
2. Simmer on low heat for 5-7 minutes. Remove from heat.
3. Add the rooibos and let steep for another 5 minutes.
4. Strain and serve with your favorite sweetener.

Iron-Rich Smoothie

PREP TIME
6 + HOURS

COOK TIME
2 MINS

SERVES
1

INGREDIENTS

1 1/2 cups water
1/4 cup raisins
1/4 cup apricots (dried)
pinch of fennel seeds
1/4" piece fresh ginger (peeled) or 1/4 teaspoon dried ginger
1 tablespoon molasses

INSTRUCTIONS

1. Soak raisins, fennel, and apricots in water for 6 hours or overnight.
2. Add all ingredients together in blender and blend until smooth.
3. Heat on the stovetop.
4. Serve warm.

Sweet & Simple Tahini Milk

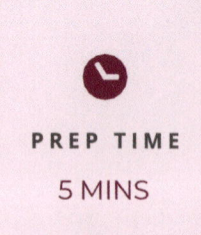

PREP TIME
5 MINS

COOK TIME
0 MINS

SERVES
2

INGREDIENTS

1 1/2 tablespoons tahini
1 1/2 tablespoons honey
2 cups hot water
dash of cinnamon
dash of cardamom

INSTRUCTIONS

1. Blend all ingredients until smooth.
2. Serve warm.

La Horchata de Mamá

PREP TIME
2 MINS

COOK TIME
0 MINS

SERVES
2-3

INGREDIENTS

3 1/2 cups hot water
1 cup basmati rice (cooked)
4 tablespoons jaggery
1" cinnamon stick or 1 teaspoon of powder
2 teaspoons ghee
1/4 teaspoon nutmeg
1/2 teaspoon vanilla extract or powder

INSTRUCTIONS

1. Add all ingredients into blender and blend on high for 2 minutes. *If you have a Vitamix or other high-power blender, add the whole cinnamon stick. If you have a regular blender, its best to use the powder.*
2. Strain and serve warm.

RejuvenDate Shake

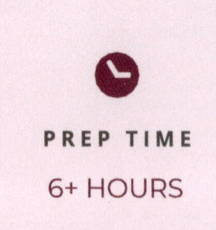

PREP TIME
6+ HOURS

COOK TIME
0 MINS

SERVES
4

INGREDIENTS

6 cups warm water
1/2 cup raw almonds
10 dates (pitted)
1/4 teaspoon cardamom powder
1/4 teaspoon fennel seeds
1 pinch saffron
1 pinch ginger powder (optional)

INSTRUCTIONS

1. Soak almonds for 6 hours or overnight.
2. Soak fennel seeds and saffron in warm water for at least 10 minutes.
3. Peel off almond skins.
4. Add all ingredients to the blender and process until smooth.
5. Serve warm.

Cream of Wheat with Ground Almonds

PREP TIME
5 MINS

COOK TIME
5 MINS

SERVES
2

INGREDIENTS

1/2 cup cream of wheat (farina)
2 cups water
1/2 cup milk
1/2 teaspoon cardamom
1/4 teaspoon ginger powder
1/8 teaspoon nutmeg powder
2 teaspoon ghee or sesame oil
3 tablespoons coconut sugar
1 tablespoon ground almonds (blanched)

INSTRUCTIONS

1. Place cream of wheat, spices, oil, water, milk, and sugar in a saucepan and bring to a boil.
2. Stir constantly to avoid lumps as the cereal thickens. Turn down heat to medium low and continue cooking for a few minutes.
3. Serve porridge in a bowl with ground almonds or almond flour sprinkled on top.

Note: To make your own ground almond flour: Soak almonds for at least 5 hours and peel off skins. If you are short on time, place the almonds in a mug and pour boiling water over them. After 5-10 minutes, drain the water and peel off the skins. Grind almonds and set aside.

Coconut Maple Tapioca Pudding

PREP TIME 30 MINS | **COOK TIME** 15 MINS | **SERVES** 2

INGREDIENTS

5 tablespoons tapioca (small pearl)
14 oz can coconut milk
1 cup water
1/2 tablespoon cardamom powder
1/3 teaspoon ginger powder
1/3 cup maple syrup
1/2 teaspoon vanilla powder or extract
shredded coconut (for garnish)

INSTRUCTIONS

1. Soak tapioca in water for 30 minutes. Drain.
2. Add tapioca, coconut milk, water, and spices to a heavily bottomed saucepan. Bring to a simmer for 15 minutes and stir periodically to avoid sticking.
3. When cooked through (if you can still see a white dot in the middle of the pearls, it is not done), turn off heat and stir in maple syrup and vanilla.
4. Garnish with coconut, and serve warm.

Note: Great recipe for your VitaClay. Add all ingredients the night before and program to be ready for you in the morning!

Replenishing Urad Dal Soup

PREP TIME
40 MINS

COOK TIME
1+ HOURS

SERVES
2-3

INGREDIENTS

1 cup white urad dal
4 cups water
1/4 teaspoon turmeric
3 tablespoons ghee or sesame oil
2 garlic cloves (minced)
1 teaspoon cumin seed
2 pinches hing (asafoetida)
1/2 tablespoon *Mama's Masala (page 46)*
1/4 teaspoon fenugreek powder
1/2 tablespoon coconut sugar
2 tablespoons cilantro (chopped)
1/2 tablespoon tamarind paste or lemon juice
1 1/2 teaspoons salt

INSTRUCTIONS

1. Soak urad dal in water for at least 30 minutes. Drain.
2. Rinse dal under warm running water until clear. Drain.
3. Add dal, water, turmeric and 1 tablespoon of ghee to a medium saucepan or VitaClay.
4. Cook until very soft and mushy. On the stovetop, about an hour. In your VitaClay 2-3 hours.
5. Heat the rest of the ghee in a medium frying pan and add the minced garlic. When the garlic starts to brown, add the cumin seed.
6. When the cumin also starts to brown, add the hing, fenugreek powder and masala. Stir until fragrant.
7. Add the sugar and cilantro and stir for a few moments until cilantro is wilted.
8. Pour the spice mixture into the soup.
9. Add tamarind paste and salt. Stir until well combined.
10. Serve hot.

Womb Rejuvenating Kitchari

PREP TIME
40 MINS

COOK TIME
1+ HOURS

SERVES
2-3

INGREDIENTS

1/3 cup yellow mung dal
2/3 cup basmati rice
3 tablespoons ghee or sesame oil
4 cups water
1/4 teaspoon turmeric
1/2 bunch of asparagus
pinch of saffron
1/2 teaspoon cumin seeds
1/8 teaspoon hing (asafoetida)
1/4 teaspoon fenugreek powder
1/2 teaspoon black pepper
Salt to taste

INSTRUCTIONS

1. Soak yellow mung dal and rice in water for at least 30 minutes. Drain.
2. Rinse rice and dal under warm running water until clear. Drain.
3. Add rice, dal, water, turmeric and 1 tablespoon of ghee to a medium saucepan or slow cooker.
4. Cook until very soft and mushy, about one hour on the stovetop or 2-3 hours in your VitaClay.
5. While kitchari is cooking, cut the more woody bottoms off the asparagus and discard, as they are hard to digest.
6. Chop the rest of the asparagus into small, bite-sized pieces.
7. Soak the saffron in a small cup of warm water.
8. Heat the rest of the ghee in a medium frying pan and add cumin seeds and hing. When the cumin starts to brown, add the fenugreek powder. Stir until fragrant.
9. Add the asparagus and stir-fry 7-10 minutes.
10. Add spiced asparagus to kitchari and cook another 10 minutes.
11. Stir in black pepper, salt and saffron and serve hot.

Mama's Mung Soup

PREP TIME
30 MINS

COOK TIME
1+ HOURS

SERVES
4

INGREDIENTS

1 cup yellow mung dal
4 cups water
1/4 teaspoon turmeric powder
3 tablespoons ghee or sesame oil
2" piece cinnamon stick
2 teaspoons cumin seeds
1/2 teaspoons fenugreek seeds
1" piece fresh ginger
1/8 teaspoon cayenne powder
2 teaspoons *Mama's Masala (pg 46)*
1 tablespoon coconut sugar
2-3 tablespoons cilantro (chopped)
1 tablespoon tamarind paste
1/2 teaspoon salt

INSTRUCTIONS

1. Soak mung dal for 30 minutes.
2. Rinse the mung dal under warm running water until clear. Drain.
3. Add dal, water, turmeric, 1 tablespoon of ghee, and the cinnamon stick to a medium saucepan or VitaClay cooker.
4. Cook until very soft and mushy, about one hour on the stovetop, or 2-3 hours in your VitaClay.
5. Add remaining oil to a small frying pan on medium heat, then add cumin. When the seeds start to brown, add fenugreek, grated ginger, sugar, cayenne, and mama's spice masala.
6. When the mixture caramelizes and turns reddish brown, add cilantro.
7. Stir and add to soup.
8. Add tamarind and salt to the soup, and serve hot.

Chai Spice Kitchari with Fennel

PREP TIME
40 MINS

COOK TIME
1+ HOURS

SERVES
2-3

INGREDIENTS

1/3 cup yellow mung dal
2/3 cup basmati rice
2 tablespoons cilantro
2 tablespoons shredded coconut
1 1/2" piece fresh ginger
8 cups water + 1/2 cup (for blending)
2" cinnamon stick
1/2 teaspoon cardamom powder
1/2 teaspoon clove powder
1/4 teaspoon turmeric powder
1/2 teaspoon black pepper
3 tablespoons ghee
1/2 fennel bulb (finely chopped)
Salt to taste

INSTRUCTIONS

1. Soak yellow mung dal for 30 minutes. Drain.
2. Wash mung dal and rice until warm running water until clear. Drain.
3. Add cilantro, coconut, ginger, and a 1/2 cup of water to a blender and blend until liquified.
4. Heat ghee on medium in a medium-sized saucepan and add blended mixture. Add the rest of the spices and sauté for 30 seconds.
5. Add rice and mung beans and fennel and sauté for another minute.
6. Add water, stir, and bring to a boil.
7. Turn down to medium-low. Cover and simmer for 1 hour or until soft.
8. Add salt and ghee as desired and serve hot.

Note: If using your VitaClay, simply add all ingredients, except salt, to the cooker and cook for 2-3 hours. Add salt and serve.

Iron-Rich Tamarind Chutney

PREP TIME
15 MINS

COOK TIME
0 MINS

SERVES
30

INGREDIENTS

1/4 teaspoon saffron
1/3 cup almond milk
2 tablespoons ghee
1 tablespoon coconut sugar
1 tablespoon tamarind paste
1/8 tsp cayenne powder
1/2 teaspoon ginger powder
6 dates (pitted)
1/8 teaspoon nutmeg powder
3/4 teaspoon cardamom powder
1 tablespoon molasses

INSTRUCTIONS

1. Soak saffron in almond milk for 10 minutes.
2. Add all ingredients to a blender, and blend till smooth.

Tasty Quinoa

PREP TIME
5 MINS

COOK TIME
25 MINS

SERVES
2

INGREDIENTS

1/2 cup quinoa
1 tablespoon ghee
1 garlic clove (minced)
1 1/4 cup water
1/4 teaspoon black pepper
1/4 teaspoon salt

INSTRUCTIONS

1. Heat ghee in small saucepan. Add minced garlic and lightly brown over medium-low heat.
2. Rinse quinoa, drain and add to the pot. Stir-fry quinoa with garlic for 1 minute.
3. Add water, salt and pepper and bring to a boil.
4. Once boiling, turn down to low heat, partially cover and cook for 20 minutes.
5. Serve hot.

Simple Postpartum Rice

PREP TIME
2 MINS

COOK TIME
25 MINS

SERVES
4

INGREDIENTS

1 cup basmati rice
1 tablespoon ghee or sesame oil
3 cups water
1/2 teaspoon black pepper
1/4 teaspoon salt

INSTRUCTIONS

1. Rinse rice under warm running water until clear. Drain.
2. Add ghee or oil to small saucepan on moderate heat.
3. Add rice and stir-fry for 1 minute.
4. Add water, salt and pepper and bring to a boil.
5. Turn down to low heat, cover and cook for 20 minutes. Do not stir.
6. Serve hot.

Butternut Squash Soup

PREP TIME
40 MINS

COOK TIME
15 MINS

SERVES
3

INGREDIENTS

1 small butternut squash (4 cups cooked)
2 1/2 cups water
1/2 cup coconut milk
1/2 teaspoon hing (asafoetida)
2 pinches nutmeg
1/2 teaspoon cinnamon powder
1 1/2 tablespoon fresh ginger (chopped)
2 tablespoons ghee or sesame oil
1/2 teaspoon black pepper
1/4 teaspoon allspice
3/4 teaspoon salt
1/2 teaspoon lemon juice

INSTRUCTIONS

1. Preheat oven to 400°F. Cut squash in half lengthwise and scoop out the seeds.
2. Add a thin layer of water to the bottom of a baking sheet and place the squash face down.
3. Cook 30-40 minutes, or until squash is soft when poked with a fork.
4. Take squash out of the oven and turn over to cool for about 5 minutes.
5. Scoop out the squash meat (discard the skin) and measure out 4 cups worth.
6. Heat ghee or oil in medium saucepan on medium heat. Fry ginger, hing, allspice and nutmeg for 1 minute.
7. Add water and squash, and simmer for 10 minutes.
8. Transfer to blender and add coconut milk, salt, pepper and lemon. juice. Blend until smooth.
9. Transfer back to the saucepan and serve hot.

Daughter's Delight Cardamom Cream

PREP TIME
10 MINS

COOK TIME
0 MINS

SERVES
4

INGREDIENTS

1 cup heavy whipping cream
2 tablespoons turbinado sugar
1/2 teaspoon cardamom powder
1/4 teaspoon vanilla extract

INSTRUCTIONS

1. Add all ingredients to a large bowl and whip with electric beaters until soft peaks form.
2. Enjoy by itself in early postpartum, or as a topping for another tasty treat such as *Divine Caramel Halva (page 66) or Yam Halva (page 68)*.

Divine Caramel Halva

PREP TIME
5 MINS

COOK TIME
20-40 MINS

SERVES
8

INGREDIENTS

4 cups cream-top milk
2 pinches saffron
1 cup wheat or rice farina
1/2 cup ghee
1 1/4 teaspoons ginger powder
1 teaspoon cardamom powder
1/4 teaspoon nutmeg powder
1/2 cup coconut sugar

INSTRUCTIONS

1. In a heavy bottomed or non-stick saucepan, bring milk to a boil. Turn off heat. Add the saffron.
2. Melt ghee in frying pan on medium heat and add farina and ginger powder.
3. Slowly brown the farina in ghee until it turns a couple of shades darker - about 10 minutes.
4. Take pan off heat for a moment and whisk in the milk until well combined.
5. Put back on medium heat and add sugar and spices.
6. Cook until the mixture thickens and pulls away from the sides of the pan. 8 minutes for wheat farina and 30 minutes for rice farina.
7. Serve warm as a pudding or pour into a 8x8 square baking dish and let cool. Cut into squares and serve at room temperature.

Note: This is truly divine salvation for new mothers (and anyone else that tastes it!)

Cardamom Vanilla Rice Pudding

PREP TIME
6+ HOURS

COOK TIME
1 HOUR

SERVES
4-6

INGREDIENTS

1/3 cup raw almonds
1 cup basmati rice
2 cups water
7 cups milk
2 tablespoons ghee
1 cup turbinado sugar
1 teaspoon cardamom powder
1 teaspoon vanilla extract or powder

INSTRUCTIONS

1. Soak almonds 6 hours, or overnight. Remove skins and thinly slice.
2. Rinse rice until water runs clear. Drain.
3. Add water and rice to medium saucepan. Bring to a boil and add milk and ghee. When it starts bubbling, turn down to a low simmer and partially cover.
4. Cook for 50 minutes, stirring frequently.
5. Add the sugar, cardamom and vanilla and continue cooking on low for 10 more minutes.
6. Remove from heat and stir in the almonds.
7. Serve hot.

Yam Halva

PREP TIME 10 MINS

COOK TIME 25 MINS

SERVES 4

INGREDIENTS

2 1/2 cups yams (grated)
4 tablespoons ghee
2 cups milk + 1 tablespoon
Pinch of saffron
1 teaspoon cardamom powder
1/2 cup dates (chopped)
1/2 cup almond flour (blanched)

INSTRUCTIONS

1. Wash, peel and grate yams.
2. Add 1 tablespoon of milk and a pinch of saffron to a cup and let soak for 10 minutes.
3. Sauté yams with ghee in medium saucepan on moderate heat for 3 minutes.
4. Stir in the saffron, milk and cardamom and bring to a boil.
5. Reduce heat to a simmer and cook covered until soft, about 25 minutes.
6. Stir in the dates and almond flour.
7. Serve warm.

Sesame Halva

PREP TIME
15 MINS

COOK TIME
0 MINS

SERVES
12

INGREDIENTS

1 1/2 cups white sesame seeds
1/2 cup raw honey
3 tablespoons ghee
1/4 teaspoon cinnamon powder
1/4 teaspoon cardamom powder

INSTRUCTIONS

1. Dry roast sesame seeds in skillet over medium heat. Stir frequently, until they turn golden brown and begin to pop.
2. Remove from stove and grind to a powder in blender or spice grinder.
3. In a medium sized bowl, mix in the honey, spices, and ghee.
4. Press into an oiled loaf pan or roll into balls.

Soothing Pear Delight

PREP TIME
7 MINS

COOK TIME
15 MINS

SERVES
2-3

INGREDIENTS

6 pears
2 cups water
2 tablespoons ghee
1/2 cup jaggery or coconut sugar
1/2 teaspoon nutmeg
2" fresh ginger
1/2 cup chopped walnuts or pecans
1/2 cup dates (pitted)

INSTRUCTIONS

1. Wash, core and chop pears into bite size pieces.
2. Add water, chopped pears, ghee, sugar and spices to a saucepan and bring to a boil.
3. Turn down to a simmer and cook with the lid off until pears are soft and the liquid has thickened, about 15 minutes.
4. Turn off stove and stir in the chopped dates and nuts.
5. Serve warm for breakfast or as a snack.

Chapter 3

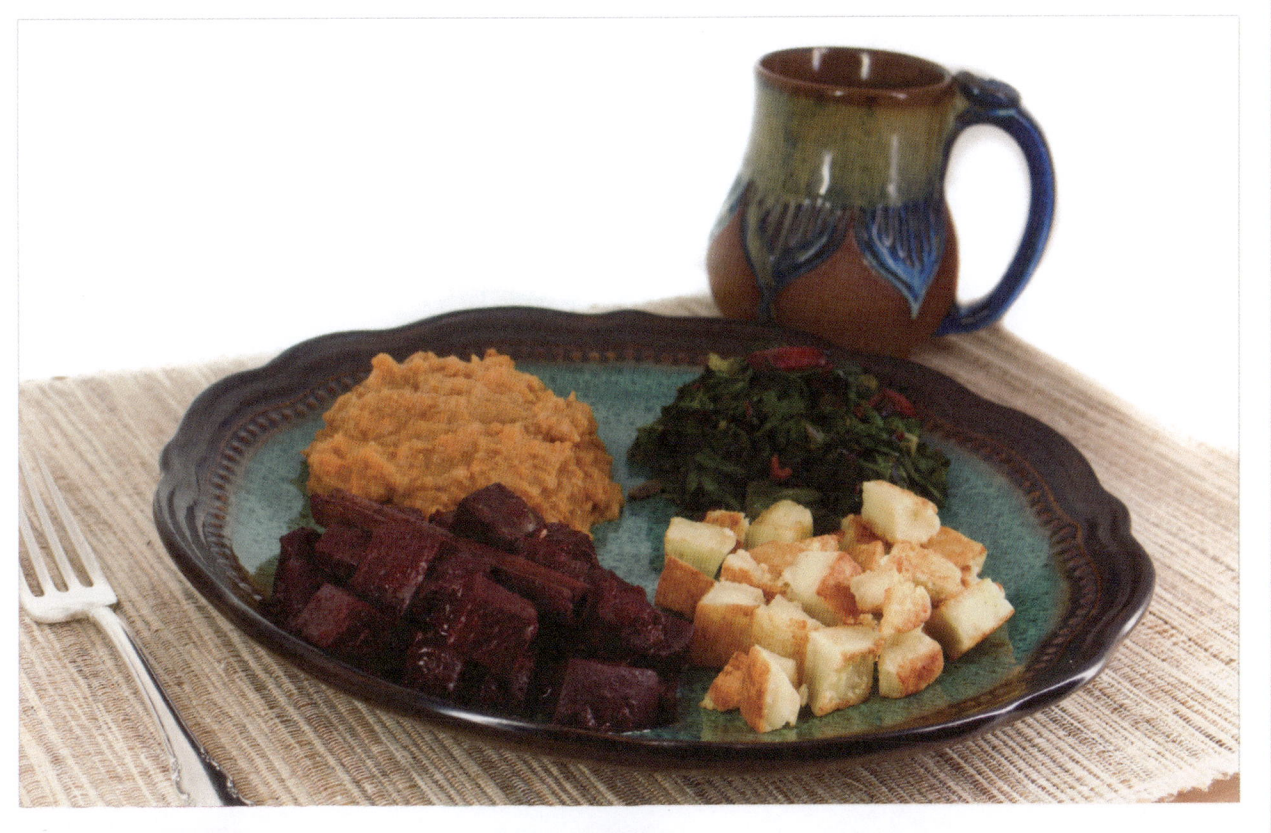

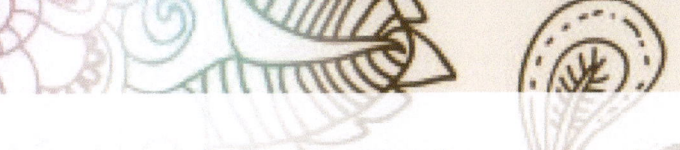

Lactation & Rejuvenation

Days 11-21

Strawberry & Cream Smoothie

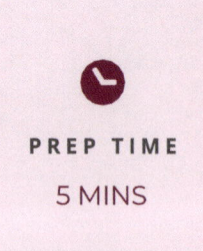

PREP TIME
5 MINS

COOK TIME
0 MINS

SERVES
2

INGREDIENTS

10 fresh strawberries
1/2 ripe banana
1/2 can of coconut milk
1 1/2 cups room temperature water
1/2" piece fresh ginger (peeled)
2 pinches of vanilla powder (optional)

INSTRUCTIONS

1. Wash and cut the tops off the strawberries.
2. Put the strawberries, banana, coconut milk, water, ginger and optional vanilla in the blender.
3. Blend until smooth and enjoy at room temperature.

Oatmeal with Crystalized Ginger

PREP TIME
5 MINS

COOK TIME
20 MINS

SERVES
2-3

INGREDIENTS

1 cup rolled oats
4 cups water
1 tablespoon ghee or unsalted butter*
1/4 cup coconut sugar or maple syrup
1/2 teaspoon cinnamon powder
1/4 cup crystalized ginger (chopped)

*Substitute sesame oil if vegan

INSTRUCTIONS

1. Add oats, water, ghee, sweetener, and cinnamon to a medium saucepan, and bring to a boil.
2. Turn down heat to medium-low and cook for 15-20 minutes. Cover as needed
3. While oatmeal is cooking, mince crystalized ginger.
4. When oatmeal is done, stir in crystalized ginger and serve hot.

Note: A great recipe for your VitaClay cooker. Add all ingredients to your VitaClay the night before and program it to be ready for you for breakfast in the morning!

Hearty Roots & Barley Stew

PREP TIME
15 MINS

COOK TIME
40+ MINS

SERVES
3

INGREDIENTS

3/4 cup beets (chopped)
1/2 cup fennel bulb (chopped)
3/4 cup carrots (chopped)
3 tablespoons pearled barley
4 cups water
3 tablespoons ghee or sesame oil
1 tablespoon fresh ginger (minced)
1 1/2 teaspoons fresh turmeric (minced) or 1/2 teaspoon powder
1/4 teaspoon hing (asafoetida)
2 tablespoons fresh basil (chopped)
1/2 teaspoon allspice powder
1/4 teaspoon black pepper
Salt to taste

INSTRUCTIONS

1. Wash and chop vegetables into bite sized pieces.
2. Rinse barley under warm water.
3. Add ghee to medium saucepan on moderate heat.
4. Add all of the spices and fry until fragrant.
5. Add the rest of the ingredients to the pot and cook for at least an hour, or until barley is very soft.
6. Salt to taste and serve hot.

Note: This is also a great recipe for your VitaClay cooker. Stew for 2-3 hours.

Creamy Beet Soup with Tarragon

PREP TIME
2+ HOURS

COOK TIME
35 MINS

SERVES
2-3

INGREDIENTS

1/4 cup cashews
2 tablespoons sesame oil
2 garlic cloves (minced)
1/4 teaspoon hing (asafoetida)
2 teaspoons dried basil
1 teaspoon dried tarragon
4 cups water
4 cups beets (chopped)
1 teaspoon black pepper
2 teaspoons lemon juice
1 1/4 teaspoon salt

INSTRUCTIONS

1. Soak cashews for 2 hours to overnight. Drain.
2. Heat oil in medium saucepan on moderate heat.
3. Add minced garlic and cook until lightly browned.
4. Add hing, basil and tarragon and fry for 30 seconds.
5. Add beets and 2 cups of water. Simmer on medium-low heat for about 30 minutes or until beets are soft.
6. Add cashews and the remaining 2 cups of water to a blender and blend on high until very smooth.
7. Strain out the cashew meal with a strainer, or cheesecloth.
8. Add cashew milk, lemon juice, salt and pepper to the soup.
9. Stir until well combined and serve hot.

Hearty Mung Bean Soup

PREP TIME
6+ HOURS

COOK TIME
1+ HOURS

SERVES
3

INGREDIENTS

1 1/2 cup whole mung beans
6 cups water
3 tablespoons ghee or sesame oil
1 carrot (sliced)
1/2 teaspoon turmeric
1/2 teaspoon black mustard seed
1/2 teaspoon cumin seed
1/2 tablespoon curry powder
1/2 tablespoon ginger root (grated)
1 teaspoon coriander powder
1/2 teaspoon black pepper
1 teaspoon salt
1 teaspoon lemon juice
1/4 cup finely chopped cilantro

INSTRUCTIONS

1. Soak whole mung beans overnight.
2. Strain and rinse mung beans under warm water until clear. Drain.
3. Add mung beans, water, 1 tablespoon of ghee, carrot and turmeric to a medium saucepan or VitaClay.
4. *On the stovetop*: bring to a boil. Turn down heat to medium, and cook partially covered for an hour. *In your VitaClay*: stew for 2-3 hours.
5. Add the rest of the ghee to a small frying pan. Heat to medium and add black mustard seeds. Once they begin to sizzle, add cumin seed. When mustard seeds begin to pop and cumin seeds brown, add them to the soup.
6. Add the grated ginger, curry powder, coriander powder and black pepper to the soup.
7. Cook for 10 more minutes.
8. Turn off heat and stir in the lemon juice, salt and chopped cilantro.
9. Serve hot.

Vegetable Coconut Curry

PREP TIME
15 MINS

COOK TIME
50 MINS

SERVES
4

INGREDIENTS

3 cups winter squash
1 1/2 cups carrots
1 1/2 cups fennel bulb
4 tablespoons ghee
2 tablespoons fresh ginger (grated)
1 cinnamon stick
1/2 teaspoon fenugreek powder
1/2 teaspoon hing (asafoetida)
2 teaspoons coconut sugar
2 teaspoons coriander powder
2 teaspoons salt
1/2 teaspoon turmeric
1 1/2 cups coconut milk
1 cup water
3 cups spinach (chopped)
1/4 cup cilantro (chopped)

INSTRUCTIONS

1. Peel winter squash, scoop out seeds and chop into bite size pieces.
2. Chop carrots and fennel into bite size pieces.
3. Heat ghee in wok or medium/large saucepan over medium heat.
4. When hot, add grated ginger and cinnamon stick.
5. Sauté until fragrant, then add hing, coriander powder, fenugreek powder and sugar.
6. When sugar caramelizes, add chopped fennel, winter squash and carrots.
7. Sauté for 3 minutes.
8. Add water, coconut milk, salt and turmeric. Stir well and cover.
9. Reduce heat and simmer for 30-40 minutes until vegetables are soft.
10. Add spinach and cilantro and cook for 5 more minutes.
11. Serve hot.

Sweet Potato & Greens

PREP TIME 10 MINS   **COOK TIME** 30 MINS   **SERVES** 4

INGREDIENTS

4 cups sweet potatoes
1 bunch of Swiss chard
3 tablespoons ghee or sesame oil
2 tablespoons ginger root (minced)
1/4 teaspoon hing (asafoetida)
1 teaspoon coriander powder
3/4 teaspoon fenugreek powder
1/4 teaspoon cinnamon powder
1 teaspoon curry powder
2 teaspoons maple syrup
1/2 cup water
1/2 teaspoon salt

INSTRUCTIONS

1. Peel and chop sweet potatoes into bite-sized pieces.
2. Chop Swiss chard into bite sized pieces as well.
3. Heat ghee in large frying pan on medium heat.
4. Add hing, ginger, coriander and fenugreek and stir until fragrant.
5. Add the rest of the ingredients and cook covered, stirring frequently, until sweet potatoes are soft, about 25-30 minutes. Add more water if necessary to prevent burning and sticking.
6. Serve hot.

Curried Beets

PREP TIME 5 MINS

COOK TIME 40 MINS

SERVES 3

INGREDIENTS

3 1/2 cups beets (chopped)
1 1/2 tablespoons ghee
1/2 can coconut milk
1/2 cup water
8 cardamom pods
1 tablespoon ginger root (minced)
2 pinches hing (asafoetida)
1" cinnamon stick
1/4 teaspoon turmeric powder
1 teaspoon garam masala
Salt to taste

INSTRUCTIONS

1. Heat ghee in medium size saucepan on medium heat.
2. Add hing and cinnamon stick and stir until fragrant.
3. Add minced ginger, garam masala and cardamom pods and fry for 30 seconds.
4. Next, add the chopped beets, water, coconut milk and turmeric.
5. Stir well, cover and simmer over medium heat until soft, about 40 minutes.
6. Salt to taste and serve warm.

Sweet Potato Mash

PREP TIME
10 MINS

COOK TIME
15 MINS

SERVES
3

INGREDIENTS

3 sweet potatoes (3 1/2 cups chopped)
3 cups water
1 tablespoon ghee
1/2 teaspoon ginger powder
1 1/2 teaspoon cinnamon powder
1/2 teaspoon black pepper
1/2 cup almond or coconut milk
1/2 teaspoon salt

INSTRUCTIONS

1. Pour water into medium saucepan and turn on high to boil.
2. Peel sweet potatoes and chop into bite size pieces. Add to the boiling water and turn down to medium high.
3. Boil 10-15 minutes until soft. Drain.
4. Return sweet potatoes back to the pot and mash.
5. Add the remaining ingredients and mix until well combined.
6. Serve hot.

Happy Baby Fennel Dish

PREP TIME
5 MINS

COOK TIME
15 MINS

SERVES
2

INGREDIENTS

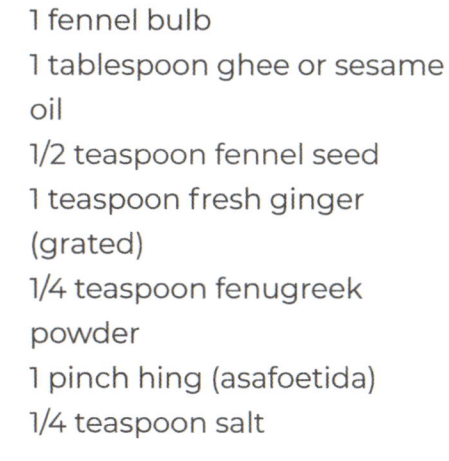

1 fennel bulb
1 tablespoon ghee or sesame oil
1/2 teaspoon fennel seed
1 teaspoon fresh ginger (grated)
1/4 teaspoon fenugreek powder
1 pinch hing (asafoetida)
1/4 teaspoon salt

INSTRUCTIONS

1. Chop the fennel into bite size pieces. Remove any woody parts.
2. Heat ghee or oil in medium frying pan on moderate heat and add fennel seed.
3. Fry until the fennel darkens a couple of shades. Add the rest of the spices and stir until fragrant.
4. Add the chopped fennel and salt, and stir fry until translucent and lightly browned, 10-15 minutes.
5. Serve hot.

Glazed Carrots

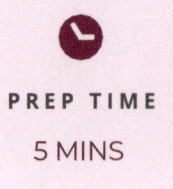

PREP TIME 5 MINS

COOK TIME 30 MINS

SERVES 2

INGREDIENTS

2 cups carrots (chopped)
1 tablespoon ghee
pinch of hing (asafoetida)
1 teaspoon fennel seeds
1/2 teaspoon cardamom powder
2 teaspoons maple syrup
1 teaspoon fresh ginger (grated)
Salt to taste

INSTRUCTIONS

1. Quarter the carrots and then chop into bite size chunks.
2. Heat ghee in small frying pan over medium heat.
3. Add hing, and let sizzle for 10 seconds. Add fennel and fry until fragrant.
4. Add grated ginger and carrots and mix well.
5. Cook over medium heat until carrots are tender, about 20-30 minutes.
6. Add cardamom, maple syrup and salt and cook a few more minutes.
7. Serve hot.

Gingered Greens

PREP TIME
5 MINS

COOK TIME
10 MINS

SERVES
2-3

INGREDIENTS

1 bunch of Swiss chard
2 tablespoons sesame oil
2 teaspoons of fresh ginger (grated)
1/2 cup water
2 teaspoons maple syrup
1/4 teaspoon salt

INSTRUCTIONS

1. Chop greens into bite sized pieces.
2. Add oil to frying pan on moderate heat.
3. Add greens, ginger and water to the pan, stir well and cover.
4. Cook for about 10 minutes, stirring occasionally, until the greens are wilted and well-cooked.
5. Add maple syrup and salt and cook for 2 more minutes.
6. Serve hot.

Fresh Paneer Cheese

PREP TIME
10+ MINS

COOK TIME
10 MINS

SERVES
2

INGREDIENTS

4 cups cream top cow milk (or goat if allergic to cow)
1 1/2 tablespoons lemon juice

INSTRUCTIONS

1. Pour milk into heavy bottomed pot (ideally ceramic non-stick). Make sure you allow room for the milk to rise to a froth.
2. Set it over high heat and bring milk to a boil. (Be careful as the foam will rise very quickly once it starts to boil).
3. Turn off heat and before the foam subsides, drizzle in the lemon juice.
4. Gently stir with a slotted spoon in a clockwise direction until the curd separates from the whey and large clumps of soft curd form.
5. Cover and set aside for 10 minutes.
6. Line a strainer with thin cotton cloth, such as cheesecloth (3 layers), a handkerchief, or a piece of thin, white cotton cloth. Make sure the corners hang over the edge.
7. Pour the contents into the strainer over the sink.
8. Rinse the curd with water.
9. Gather 2 opposing corners of the cloth and tie into a double knot.
10. Repeat with the other 2 corners.
11. Hang over the faucet in the sink to drain (around 3 hours), or to speed up the process, press over strainer with something heavy for 1 hour.
12. If you want to crumble it over your food, there is no need for step #11.

Sag Paneer

PREP TIME
5 MINS

COOK TIME
25 MINS

SERVES
2-3

INGREDIENTS

4 oz fresh paneer cheese (pg 84)
4 tablespoons ghee or sesame oil
1 1/2 teaspoon coriander powder
1 teaspoon *Mama's Masala (pg 46)* or garam masala
1/4 teaspoon nutmeg powder
1/4 teaspoon turmeric powder
1/4 teaspoon black pepper
1/8 teaspoon cayenne
3 tablespoons water
1/4 teaspoon hing (asafoetida)
2 lbs baby spinach
1 teaspoon salt
2 tablespoons goat chèvre

INSTRUCTIONS

1. Cut paneer into bite sized cubes. Heat ghee or oil to medium heat in a large frying pan and add paneer.
2. Carefully brown on each side for a few minutes, turning them each with a fork.
3. When the paneer is finished cooking, remove from pan with a slotted spoon.
4. Mix coriander, masala, turmeric, cayenne, nutmeg and black pepper together in a small cup with the 3 tablespoons of water.
5. Add hing to frying pan, fry for 10 seconds and add the spice mixture.
6. Cook spice mixture for 1 minute and add the spinach.
7. Cover and let cook on moderate heat for 1 minute, until the volume of spinach goes down.
8. Stir well, sprinkle more water if needed to prevent sticking, and cook covered for 5-7 minutes.
9. Add the spiced spinach to a blender with the goat cheese and salt.
10. Blend well.
11. Pour into a bowl and mix in the fresh Paneer.
12. Serve hot.

Vegan Lactation Pesto

PREP TIME
5 MINS

COOK TIME
5 MINS

SERVES
8

INGREDIENTS

2 cups fresh basil
1/2 cup sesame oil
3 garlic cloves (minced)
1/4 cup sesame seeds
1 teaspoon salt

INSTRUCTIONS

1. Heat 1 tablespoon of oil in frying pan on moderate heat. Add minced garlic and slowly fry in oil until the garlic is light brown in color.
2. Add all the ingredients to a blender and process until smooth.
3. If not already adding the pesto to a recipe that requires cooking, put the pesto into the frying pan and cook for 2 minutes on medium heat.

Mother's Guacamole

PREP TIME
3 MINS

COOK TIME
5 MINS

SERVES
2-3

INGREDIENTS

2 avocados (ripe)
1 tablespoon sesame oil
1 garlic clove (minced)
1 teaspoon cumin powder
1 teaspoon lemon juice
1/2 teaspoon salt
ground black pepper
(to taste)

INSTRUCTIONS

1. Cut avocados in half and take out the pit. Scoop out the flesh into a bowl. Mash avocado with a masher or fork.
2. In a small frying pan, bring sesame oil to moderate heat. Add minced garlic.
3. Sauté garlic in oil until golden brown.
4. Add cumin powder and stir until fragrant.
5. Add garlic and cumin to the mashed avocado.
6. Add the rest of the ingredients and stir until well combined.

Avocado Chutney with Crystalized Ginger

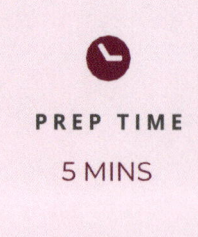

PREP TIME
5 MINS

COOK TIME
0 MINS

SERVES
2-3

INGREDIENTS

1 avocado
2 tablespoons lime juice
2 tablespoons crystallized ginger (finely chopped)
3 tablespoons pecans (chopped)
2 teaspoons honey
salt to taste

INSTRUCTIONS

1. Cut open the avocado lengthwise, remove the pit and scoop out the flesh into a bowl. Mash.
2. Add lemon juice, chopped crystalized ginger, pecans and honey. Stir until well combined.
3. Add salt and serve fresh.

Cumin Chapati Flatbread

PREP TIME 40 MINS

COOK TIME 20 MINS

SERVES 4

INGREDIENTS

1 cup whole wheat pastry flour
1 tablespoon ghee
1 teaspoon cumin seeds
1/2 cup water
1/4 teaspoon salt
extra ghee for coating

INSTRUCTIONS

1. Add flour in a bowl with ghee and cut with a pastry cutter or mix with a fork until uniformly crumbly.
2. Heat cast-iron or other frying pan on medium heat and add cumin seeds.
3. Dry roast until seeds darken a shade or two.
4. Add seeds to flour mixture.
5. Slowly add water while mixing until the flour mixture pulls away from the sides of the bowl and forms a ball.
6. Sprinkle flour onto a cutting board or other clean surface and knead dough for 8 minutes, adding more flour if it starts getting sticky.
7. Coat dough ball in a thin film of ghee and let sit for at least 30 minutes.
8. Separate dough ball into 4 equal portions and roll out dough into 6" circles.
9. Heat large cast-iron pan on medium heat. Put rolled out chapatti in pan.
10. Let cook until air bubbles form in the dough, around 3 minutes.
11. Flip over with a spatula and cook until more air bubbles form in the chapatti and it looks cooked through.
12. Flip it over 1 more time for about 30 seconds and see if any more air bubbles pop up.
13. Remove from pan, coat with ghee and repeat.

Garlic Farinata

PREP TIME
10 MINS

COOK TIME
20 MINS

SERVES
8

INGREDIENTS

1 cup garbanzo bean flour
1 1/2 cup warm water
4 tablespoons ghee
1 tablespoon garlic (minced)
2 tablespoons fresh basil (chopped)
1 teaspoon salt

INSTRUCTIONS

1. Preheat oven to 500° F.
2. Whisk garbanzo flour and warm water in a medium sized bowl till smooth. Set aside.
3. Add 1 tablespoon of ghee and minced garlic to frying pan and slowly brown on medium-low heat.
4. Add the browned garlic, salt, 2 more tablespoons of ghee, and basil to the bowl and whisk until well combined.
5. Add 1 tablespoon of ghee to a 12" cast iron skillet, put on high heat until it begins to smoke. Turn off heat.
6. Immediately pour the batter into the skillet.
7. Transfer to preheated oven immediately, and bake for 20 minutes, or until golden brown.
8. Remove from oven and let cool.

Snacking Almonds

PREP TIME
OVERNIGHT

COOK TIME
10-15 MINS

SERVES
6

INGREDIENTS

1 cup almonds
1 tablespoon ghee
3/4 teaspoon salt
3/4 teaspoon black pepper

INSTRUCTIONS

1. Soak almonds overnight.
2. Peel the skins off of the almonds and discard.
3. Add ghee to a medium frying pan and melt on medium heat.
4. When ghee is melted, add the almonds.
5. Once they begin to sizzle, turn down heat to medium-low and stir frequently to brown evenly.
6. Add salt and pepper.
7. Cook for 10-15 minutes until lightly browned.
8. Serve warm or room temperature.

Mother's Mexican Wedding Cookies

PREP TIME
15 MINS

COOK TIME
7—9 MINS

SERVES
12

INGREDIENTS

2 cups almond flour
1 pinch salt
1/2 cup toasted pecans (finely chopped)
1/2 teaspoon cinnamon powder
1/2 teaspoon vanilla powder
4 tablespoons ghee
2 tablespoons maple syrup
Cinnamon powder for garnish

INSTRUCTIONS

1. Preheat oven to 350° and line a baking tray with parchment paper.
2. Mix dry ingredients together in medium-sized bowl. Add ghee and maple syrup and mix well.
3. Scoop using a tablespoon, and form dough into a firm ball with your hands.
4. Bake 7-9 minutes.
5. Sprinkle cinnamon powder on top of the cookies.
6. Let cool for 15 minutes before serving.

Iron-Rich Ginger Cookies

PREP TIME
15 MINS

COOK TIME
10 MINS

SERVES
24

INGREDIENTS

1/2 cup ghee (softened)
1/2 cup maple syrup
1/2 cup molasses
1 tablespoon garbanzo bean flour
1 tablespoon water
2 teaspoons ginger powder
1 1/2 teaspoons cinnamon powder
2 1/4 cups whole wheat pastry flour*
1/2 teaspoon salt

*For Gluten Free Cookies replace wheat flour with:
1 cup rice flour + 1 1/2 cups oat flour

INSTRUCTIONS

1. Preheat oven to 375°.
2. Cream together ghee, maple syrup and molasses with electric beaters.
3. In a small cup whisk the garbanzo flour and water together until well combined.
4. Add garbanzo mixture and spices to the ghee mixture and cream together until well combined.
5. Add flour and salt and stir until combined with a wooden spoon.
6. Scoop using a tablespoon onto a greased cookie sheet. Make sure there is space for the cookies to expand.
7. Bake for 10 minutes or until the cookies brown around the edges.
8. Remove cookies and place on a wire rack to cool.

Chapter 4

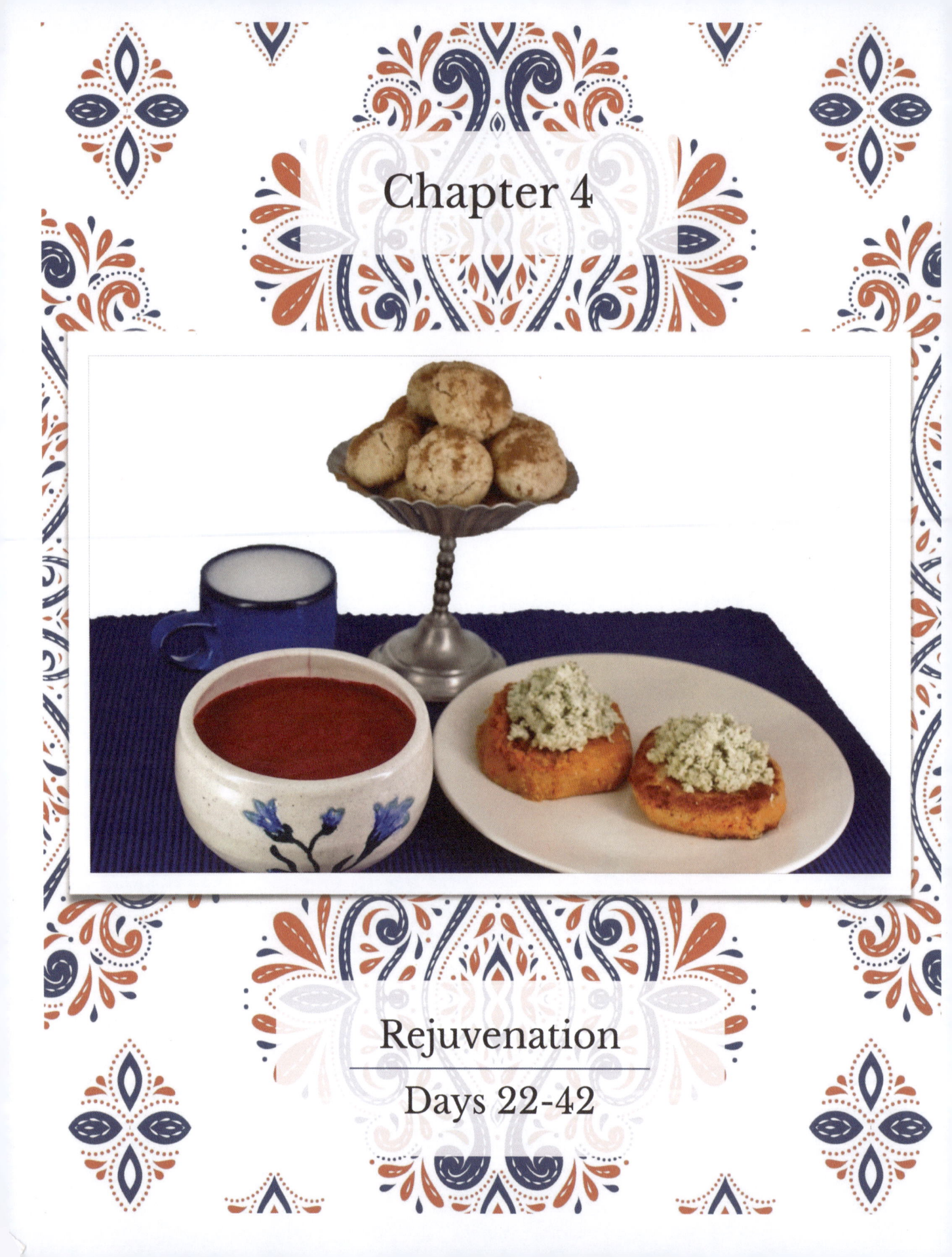

Rejuvenation

Days 22-42

Sesame Ginger-Snap Amaranth

PREP TIME
OVERNIGHT

COOK TIME
30 MINS

SERVES
2-3

INGREDIENTS

1 cup amaranth
3 cups water
3 tablespoons ghee or sesame oil
1/3 teaspoon clove powder
1/2 teaspoon ginger powder
1/3 teaspoon cinnamon powder
2 tablespoons molasses
2 tablespoons coconut sugar
1/4 cup sesame seeds (ground)

INSTRUCTIONS

1. Soak amaranth in water overnight. Drain.
2. In a small saucepan, bring amaranth, oil, and water to boil.
3. Reduce to a simmer, cover and cook for 20 minutes.
4. Add spices and molasses. Cook another 10 minutes or until soft.
5. Garnish with ground sesame seeds and serve warm.

Note: This is a great recipe for you VitaClay cooker. Add all ingredients to your VitaClay the night before, and program it to be ready for you in the morning for breakfast.

Toor Dal Soup with Pumpkin

PREP TIME 3 HOURS

COOK TIME 35 MINS

SERVES 3

INGREDIENTS

2/3 cup toor dal
4 cups water
2 cups pumpkin (peeled and chopped)
1 teaspoon fresh ginger (minced)
1/4 teaspoon turmeric
3 tablespoons ghee or sesame oil
1 teaspoon cumin seeds
1 teaspoon black mustard seeds
1/4 teaspoon fenugreek seeds
1/8 teaspoon hing (asafoetida)
1 tablespoon coconut sugar
1 1/2 teaspoons lemon juice
1 teaspoon salt
1/4 cup cilantro (chopped)

INSTRUCTIONS

1. Rinse toor dal under warm running water until clear. Soak dal in 4 cups of water for 30 minutes. Drain.
2. Add 4 cups of water, dal, pumpkin, ginger, turmeric and 1 tablespoon of ghee or oil to a pressure cooker. Cook under pressure for 30 minutes. Alternately, stew in your VitaClay for 5 hours.
3. After dal is finished cooking, heat a frying pan over moderate heat. Add the remainder of the ghee or oil.
4. Add black mustard seeds. After 30 seconds add cumin and fenugreek.
5. Once the mustard seeds begin to pop, add hing, cayenne and coconut sugar. When mixture becomes reddish brown and caramelizes, immediately add to the soup.
6. Add salt, lemon juice and chopped cilantro. Stir well.
7. Sit for 5 minutes before serving to allow the flavors to mingle.

Black Bean Soup

PREP TIME
OVERNIGHT

COOK TIME
3+ HOURS

SERVES
5

INGREDIENTS

2 cups black beans (dried)
5 cups water
1/2 cup fennel bulb (chopped)
1 carrot (sliced)
3 tablespoons sesame oil
3 garlic cloves (minced)
2 teaspoons cumin powder
2 teaspoons coriander powder
1/2 teaspoon hing (asafoetida)
1/4 teaspoon cayenne
1/2 teaspoon black pepper
1/3 cup cilantro (chopped)
2 1/4 teaspoons salt
Avocado Slices (optional)
Coconut cream (optional)

INSTRUCTIONS

1. Soak beans overnight and drain. Rinse well.
2. Add beans, water, carrot, fennel bulb and 1 tablespoon of oil to a pressure cooker or your VitaClay.
3. Cook under pressure for 30 minutes, or 3 hours in your VitaClay, until quite soft.
4. Heat the remaining 2 tablespoons of oil in a small frying pan on moderate heat. Add garlic and turn down to medium-low heat to slowly brown.
5. When lightly browned, add cumin, coriander and hing and stir until fragrant.
6. Add cayenne, black pepper, and cilantro, stir and take off heat.
7. Add spice mixture and salt to the beans and stir well.
8. Add all of the contents to a blender and blend until combined.
9. Serve hot with sliced avocado and a drizzle of coconut cream.

Oh Baby "Baked" Beans

PREP TIME
OVERNIGHT

COOK TIME
45+ MINS

SERVES
5-6

INGREDIENTS

2 1/4 cups great northern beans
3 tablespoons ghee or sesame oil
3 cups water
3" cinnamon stick
1/4 cup molasses
1/3 cup maple syrup
2 garlic cloves (minced)
1/2 teaspoon clove powder
1/4 teaspoon hing (asafoetida)
3 tablespoons arrowroot starch
6 tablespoons water (cold)
1 teaspoon salt

INSTRUCTIONS

1. Soak beans in a generous amount of water overnight. Drain and rinse.
2. Add 1 tablespoon of ghee or oil to a small frying pan on moderate heat.
3. Add minced garlic and slowly brown, turning down to medium-low once it begins to sizzle.
4. When garlic darkens a few shades, add hing and take off heat.
5. Add beans, water, garlic mixture, the cinnamon stick, 2 tablespoons of ghee or oil, molasses, maple syrup and clove powder to a pressure cooker or VitaClay. Cook under pressure for 45 minutes or stew for 5 hours in your VitaClay (preferred).
6. Mix arrowroot with cold water until well combined.
7. Add arrowroot mixture to the beans, as well as salt and stir until well combined.
8. Cook an additional 5 minutes until thick.
9. Serve hot.

I grew up in New England where baked beans is a traditional food. I loved them as a kid, and when I was pregnant, I craved them like crazy!

Pesto Sweet Potato Fries

PREP TIME
10 MINS

COOK TIME
40 MINS

SERVES
4

INGREDIENTS

2 medium sweet potatoes (about 4 1/2 cups)
1/4 cup *Vegan Lactation Pesto (page 86)*
1/2 teaspoon black pepper

INSTRUCTIONS

1. Heat the oven to 400°F.
2. Peel sweet potatoes and cut into fries 1/2'" thick and 2" long.
3. Put in a large bowl and mix in the pesto and black pepper.
4. Spread out on cookie sheet and bake for 30-40 minutes, turning the fries halfway through so they cook evenly.
5. Take out of the oven when soft and brown.

Chana Dal Hummus

PREP TIME
OVERNIGHT

COOK TIME
3+ HOURS

SERVES
8

INGREDIENTS

1 cup chana dal (split chickpeas)
3 cups water
2 tablespoons sesame oil
2 tablespoons tahini
2 garlic cloves (minced)
1 teaspoon cumin seed
1 teaspoon salt
2 tablespoons lemon juice
1/4 cup sesame seeds

INSTRUCTIONS

1. Rinse chana dal under warm running water until clear. Soak overnight, then drain.
2. Add chana dal, water and 1 tablespoon of sesame oil to your VitaClay and stew for 3 hours, or 6 hours in a regular crockpot.
3. Drain and save 1/2 cup of cooking liquid.
4. Add 2 tablespoons of sesame oil to a frying pan and slowly brown the minced garlic on medium-low. Remove garlic from the pan with a slotted spoon.
5. Add the sesame seeds and repeat.
6. Add all ingredients except the sesame seeds to a blender.
7. Blend until well combined.
8. Scoop out into a bowl and garnish with sesame seeds and a drizzle of sesame oil.
9. Serve warm with *Cumin Chapati Flatbread (page 89)*.

Garden Pasta with Pesto & Cheese

PREP TIME
15 MINS

COOK TIME
30 MINS

SERVES
4

INGREDIENTS

3 tablespoons ghee
2 cloves garlic (minced)
2 cups butternut squash (peeled and chopped)
1 1/2 cups carrots (quartered and chopped)
4 cups baby spinach
1 - 8 oz package of semolina or quinoa pasta
1/4 cup *Vegan Lactation Pesto (pg 86)*
Fresh paneer (pg 84) or goat chèvre to taste
Salt to taste

INSTRUCTIONS

1. Heat ghee in large saucepan. Add garlic and lightly brown on medium low.
2. Add the chopped butternut squash and carrots, and cook covered for 25-30 minutes, or until soft. Stir frequently.
3. Add the spinach and cook for 5 more minutes.
4. Meanwhile, cook the pasta. Follow the directions provided on the package. Drain and return pasta to the pot.
5. Mix the pesto in with the pasta until well combined.
6. Serve the vegetables on top of the pesto pasta.
7. Crumble the fresh cheese on top.
8. Salt to taste.
9. Enjoy!

Delicious Yam Patties

PREP TIME 15 MINS

COOK TIME 1 HOUR

SERVES 4

INGREDIENTS

3 medium yams
3 tablespoons almond flour
3 tablespoons sesame seeds (ground)
3 tablespoons shredded coconut
1 pinch cayenne
1 teaspoon cumin powder
1 teaspoon coriander powder
1 tablespoon coconut sugar
1 teaspoon salt
1 tablespoon arrowroot starch
1/2 cup almond flour (for coating patties)
1 tablespoon ghee

INSTRUCTIONS

1. Wash yams throughly. Add yams to boiling water and cook for 20 minutes, or until soft when pierced with a fork.
2. Drain, and peel while still warm.
3. In a large bowl, mash the yams.
4. Add 3 tablespoons of almond flour, sesame seeds, coconut, spices, sugar, salt and arrowroot. Mix until well combined.
5. Place 1/2 cup of almond flour in a shallow bowl.
6. Divide yam mixture into 6 portions.
7. Coat your hands in a thin film of ghee or oil and form each portion into a patty between your palms.
8. Coat both sides of each patty in almond flour.
9. Heat medium skillet over medium heat and add 1 tablespoon of ghee.
10. Cook until brown, 5-7 minutes on each side.
11. Serve hot.

Note: Serve with *Iron-Rich Tamarind Chutney* (page 61) and/or *Coconut Mint Chutney* (page 103).

Coconut Mint Chutney

PREP TIME
10 MINS

COOK TIME
0 MINS

SERVES
6

INGREDIENTS

2 1/4" fresh ginger
6 tablespoons fresh mint
1 cup fresh coconut meat or dried shredded coconut
10 cashews
1/3 cup water
1/4 teaspoon black pepper
1 pinch cayenne
2 tablespoons lime juice
1 tablespoon maple syrup
1 teaspoon salt

INSTRUCTIONS

1. Peel the ginger and chop into large pieces.
2. Wash the mint.
3. Add all ingredients to the blender and blend until smooth.

Note: Perfect for a hot summer day. This more cooling recipe is a delicious topping for Delicious Yam Patties (pg 102). Only eat this chutney between 21-42 days when your digestive fire is strong.

Black Bean Croquets

PREP TIME
OVERNIGHT

COOK TIME
3+ HOURS

SERVES
3

INGREDIENTS

1 cup dried black beans
6 cups water
3 tablespoons sesame oil
1 cup quinoa (cooked)
1/3 cup fennel bulb (chopped fine)
1 cup carrot (finely grated)
2 garlic cloves (minced)
3 tablespoons ghee or sesame oil
1 teaspoon cumin seed
1/2 teaspoon coriander powder
1 teaspoon salt
2/3 cup almond flour
Sesame oil for frying

INSTRUCTIONS

1. Soak black beans in water overnight. Drain and rinse.
2. Add beans, water, and 1 tablespoon of oil to a pressure cooker or VitaClay. Cook under pressure for 30 minutes or stew in a VitaClay for 3 hours.
3. Add beans to a blender, adding just enough water to blend them thoroughly. Cool enough to handle.
4. Heat oil to moderate in a medium skillet and add minced garlic, cumin, and coriander. Fry until garlic is lightly browned.
5. Add chopped fennel and grated carrot and cook 7-10 minutes, or until soft.
6. In a large bowl mix the beans, vegetables, almond flour, salt, and quinoa.
7. Shape the mixture into patties.
8. Add sesame oil to a non-stick skillet. Fry the croquets on both sides until golden brown.

Note: Delicious with Avocado Chutney with Crystalized Ginger (page 88)

Vegetable Koorma with Fennel

PREP TIME
15 MINS

COOK TIME
25 MINS

SERVES
4

INGREDIENTS

1 tablespoon fennel seeds
10 clove buds
1/2 teaspoon cardamom seeds
1/2 teaspoon cinnamon powder
1/4 teaspoon cayenne
4 tablespoons ghee
1 1/2 cups fennel bulb (chopped)
1 1/2 cups carrot (sliced)
2 1/2 cups zucchini (quartered and chopped)
1 cup almond flour
1 1/4" fresh ginger (peeled)
1 cup coconut milk
1 cup water
2 teaspoons coconut sugar
2 teaspoons salt

INSTRUCTIONS

1. In a cast iron skillet on moderate heat, dry roast fennel, cardamom and clove until fragrant.
2. Grind spices with an electric grinder or mortar and pestle. Add cinnamon and cayenne powder to mixture and set aside.
3. Add ghee to a large skillet on medium heat. Add fennel and carrot, stir, partially cover and cook for 5 minutes.
4. Add zucchini, stir well and continue cooking, partially covered for 5 more minutes.
5. In a blender, add almond flour, coconut milk, water, fresh ginger, spice mixture, salt and sugar. Blend until smooth.
6. Add contents of blender to the vegetables, turn down heat to medium low, stir well and cover.
7. Cook for 10-15 minutes, stirring occasionally.
8. Serve hot.

Curried Black Bean & Sweet Potato Burrito

PREP TIME
OVERNIGHT

COOK TIME
50+ MINS

SERVES
4

INGREDIENTS

1 cup black beans
2 cups water
3 tablespoons ghee
2 recipes of *Cumin Chapatti Flatbread (pg 89)*
2 sweet potatoes (small)
3 cups baby spinach
2 garlic cloves (minced)
1 teaspoon curry powder
1/2 teaspoon cumin seed
1/4 teaspoon cinnamon powder
1/2 teaspoon salt

Optional - avocado or Mother's Guacamole (pg 87)
Fresh Paneer (pg 84)

INSTRUCTIONS

1. Soak beans overnight. Drain and rinse.
2. Add beans, water and 1 tablespoon of ghee to a pressure cooker or VitaClay. Cook under pressure for 30 minutes or 3 hours in your VitaClay. Drain.
3. Make the dough for the *Cumin Chapatti Flatbread* recipe. Instead of separating the dough into quarters, separate it into halves.
4. Preheat the oven to 400°F.
5. Wash sweet potatoes and poke 4+ times with a fork. When oven is up to temperature, put the sweet potatoes in.
6. Cook for 40 minutes or until soft when poked with a fork.
7. Cut lengthwise and scoop the flesh out of the skin (discard skin).
8. Heat remaining ghee or oil in medium frying pan to a moderate temperature.
9. Add minced garlic and cook until brown. Add cumin seed and cook until fragrant.
10. Add sweet potato and beans, spinach, salt, curry and cinnamon powders and stir until well combined. Add a sprinkling of water to prevent sticking and cook covered for 5 minutes.
11. Roll out the chapati dough into two 12" rounds and cook as instructed in recipe.
12. Scoop bean/potato filling into the chapatti, add optional avo/guac and paneer and devour!

Postnatal Pad Thai

PREP TIME
10 MINS

COOK TIME
30 MINS

SERVES
3

INGREDIENTS

8 oz pad thai rice noodles
8 oz sprouted tofu or *Fresh Paneer (pg 84)*
4 tablespoons sesame oil
2 garlic cloves (minced)
1 cup fennel bulb (chopped)
1/4 teaspoon hing (asafoetida)
1 1/4 cup sugar snap peas
9 oz mung sprouts
1 tablespoon tamarind paste
2 teaspoons coconut sugar
3 tablespoons coconut aminos (avoid soy sauce)
1/8 teaspoon cayenne
2 tablespoons water
1 1/2 teaspoons lime juice
1/2 cup roasted cashews
1 tablespoon sesame oil

INSTRUCTIONS

1. Cook noodles per instructions provided on the package. Drain.
2. Cut tofu or paneer into cubes.
3. Heat a large skillet on moderate heat. Add 3 tablespoons of sesame oil and the tofu/paneer.
4. Fry for a few minutes on each side, turning to brown evenly. Remove with a slotted spoon.
5. Add garlic and turn down the heat to medium low. Slowly brown for 3-5 minutes.
6. Add chopped fennel and hing and turn up heat to moderate. Cook until translucent, about 10 minutes.
7. Add peas and mung sprouts and sauté for 3 minutes.
8. In a small cup, mix tamarind paste, coconut sugar, coconut aminos, and cayenne with 2 tablespoons of water.
9. Add the noodles and the tamarind mixture, and stir well. Cook for another 5 minutes, stirring frequently to prevent sticking. Stir in the lime juice.
10. Heat 1 tablespoon of sesame oil in a small frying pan on medium low heat. Add cashews and sprinkle with salt. Fry until golden brown.
11. Top the dish with tofu/paneer and cashews. Serve hot.

Fig Crescents

PREP TIME
75 MINS

COOK TIME
30 MINS

SERVES
16

INGREDIENTS

1 1/4 cups whole wheat pastry flour
1/2 cup ghee or butter
1/4 teaspoon salt
1/3 cup *Fresh Paneer (pg 84)*
3 tablespoons yogurt
1/2 cup dates (chopped)
4 tablespoons coconut sugar
4 tablespoons fig jam
1/2 cup pecans (ground)
1 tablespoon cinnamon powder

INSTRUCTIONS

To make the dough:
1. Add flour, ghee, salt, paneer and yogurt to a food processor fitted with a metal blade.
2. Pulse about 15 times until well combined.
3. Form into a ball, then flatten into a thick round.
4. Wrap in plastic and refrigerate for 1 hour.

To make the filling:
1. Mix chopped dates, pecans, coconut sugar, fig jam and cinnamon powder until well combined.

To assemble the crescents:
1. Cover a cookie sheet with parchment paper and pre-heat oven to 350° F.
2. Pull the dough out of the refrigerator, unwrap and cut in half with a sharp knife.
3. Sprinkle flour on a smooth surface and roll out the first half of the dough into a 10" round.
4. Evenly spread half of the filling onto the dough and then cut into 8 wedges (Like a pizza).
5. Roll each wedge unto itself, starting with the widest part first and finishing with the points.
6. Fold in the corners to shape it into a crescent.
7. Repeat process with the other half of ingredients.
8. Bake for 30 minutes or until golden brown.

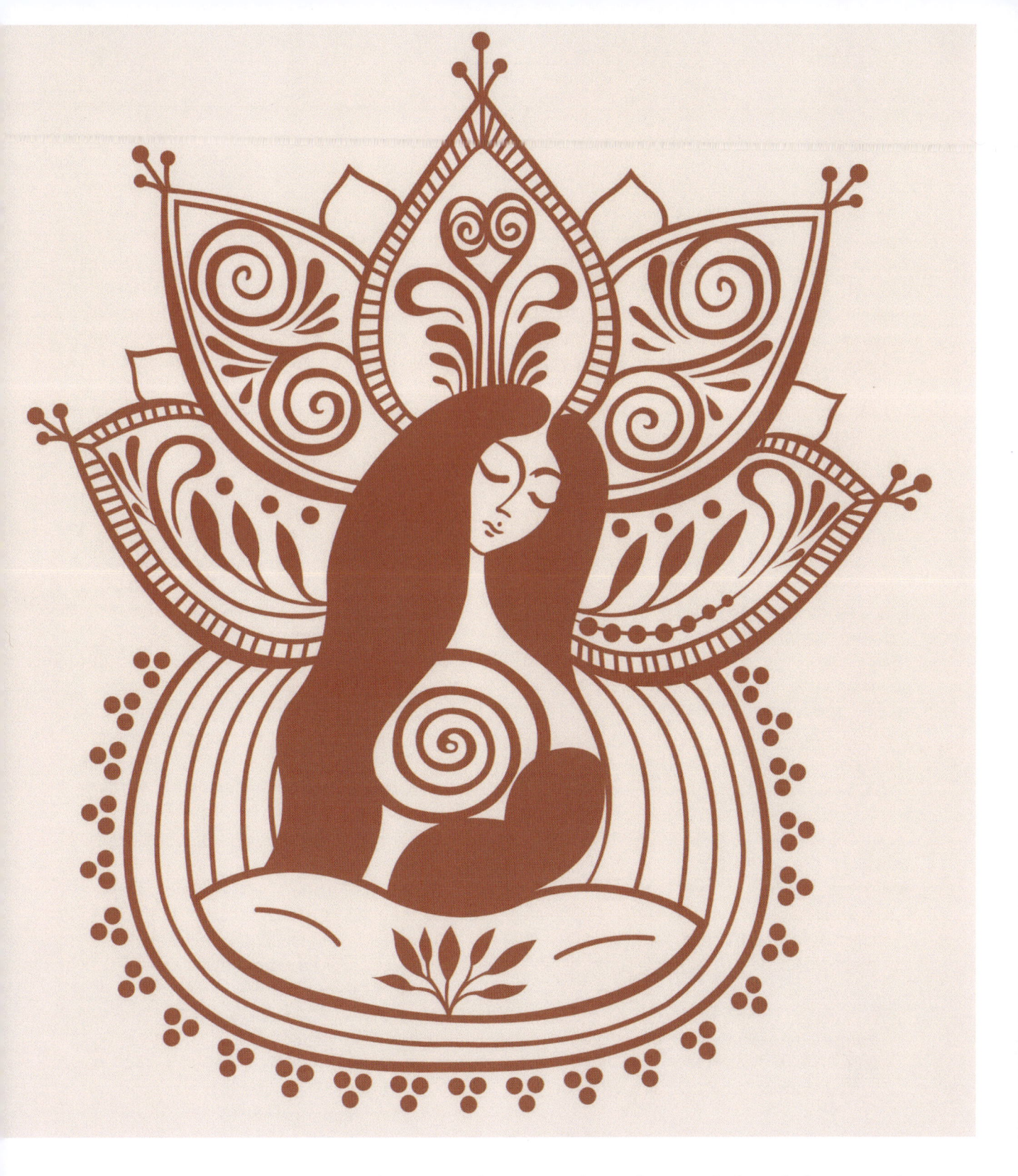

May your journey through motherhood be blessed.

Index

Agni 21
Ajwain seeds 24, 31, 43
Alcohol 25
Allspice 24, 31, 64, 74
Almonds 23, 24, 31
    Flour (Blanched) 40, 44, 45, 55, 68, 92, 102, 104, 105
    Milk 50, 61, 80
    Whole (Raw) 44, 54, 55, 67, 91
Amaranth 24, 31, 95
Apples 32, 45
Apricots (Dried) 32, 51
Arrowroot starch 31, 98, 102
Asafoetida (Hing) 24, 31, 33, 57, 58, 64, 74, 75, 77 - 79, 81, 82, 85, 96-98, 107
Avocado 32, 87, 88, 97, 104, 106
Bananas 32, 72
Baked Beans 98
Basil 24, 31, 74, 75, 86, 90
Barley 31, 74
Beets 32, 74, 75, 79
Black beans 32, 97, 104, 106
Black mustard seed 31, 76, 96
Black Pepper 24, 31, 37-39, 43, 46, 50, 58, 60, 62-64, 74-76, 80, 85, 87, 91, 97, 99, 103
Brassicas see Cruciferous
Breakfast
    Coconut Maple Tapioca Pudding 56
    Cream of Rice with Dates 41
    Cream of Wheat with Ground Almonds 55
    First Days Rice Congee 37
    Rabb 40
    Sesame Ginger-Snap Amaranth 95
    Soothing Pear Delight 70
    Toasted Oatmeal with Crystalized Ginger 73
Breads
    Cumin Chapati Flatbread 89
    Garlic Farinata 90
Butter 24, 31, 37, 47, 73, 108

Butternut squash 32, 64, 101
Caffeine 25
Carbonated beverages 25
Cardamom 24, 31, 33, 37, 38, 44, 46, 50, 52, 54-56, 60, 61, 65 - 69, 79, 82, 105
Carrots 32, 74, 77, 82, 101
Cashews 23, 31, 75, 103, 107
Cayenne 20, 24, 31, 37, 42, 59, 61, 85, 96, 97, 102, 103, 105, 107
Chana dal 32, 33, 100
Chocolate 25
Cilantro 32, 43, 57, 59, 60, 76, 77, 96, 97
Cinnamon 24, 31, 37, 41, 45, 46, 50, 52, 53, 59, 60, 64, 69, 73, 77-80, 92, 93, 95, 98, 105, 106, 108
Cloves 24, 31
    Whole 38, 50, 105
    Powder 37, 41 - 43, 45, 46, 60, 95, 98
Coconut 24, 31, 32
    Aminos 33, 107
    Milk (see *Milk*)
    Shredded 39, 43, 46, 56, 60, 102, 103
    Sugar (see *Sugar*)
Cold foods 25
Condiments
    Avocado Chutney with Crystalized Ginger 88
    Chana Dal Hummus 100
    Coconut Mint Chutney 103
    Daughter's Delight Cardamom Cream 65
    Iron-Rich Tamarind Chutney 61
    Mother's Guacamole 87
    Vegan Lactation Pesto 86
    Vital Garlic Chutney 39
Coriander powder 31, 39, 46, 76-78, 85, 97, 102, 104
Cream of wheat (farina) 31, 55
Cruciferous vegetables 25
Cumin 24, 31, 42, 43, 46, 57-59, 76, 87, 89, 96, 97, 100, 102, 104, 106
Curry powder 31, 76, 78, 106

Dates   23, 24, 32, 41, 54, 61, 68, 70, 108
Desserts
    Almond Kheer   44
    Cardamom Vanilla Rice Pudding   67
    Divine Carmel Halva   66   Fig Crescents   108
    Iron-Rich Ginger Cookies   93
    Mother's Mexican Wedding Cookies   92
    Sesame Halva   69
    Yam Halva   68
Doshas (Constitution - Vata, Pitta, Kapha)   14, 15, 27, 28
Dry foods   25
Drinks
    Milks
        La Horchata de Mamá   53
        Mother's Milk   38
        Sweet & Simple Tahini Milk   52
    Smoothies
        Iron-Rich Smoothie   51
        RejuvenDate Shake   54
        Strawberry & Cream Smoothie   72
    Teas
        Mother's Red Chai   50
        Simple Lactation Tea   49
        Strong Fenugreek Tea   36
Fennel
    Bulb   24, 32, 60, 74, 77, 81, 97, 104, 105, 107
    Seed   24, 31, 38, 46, 49 - 51, 54, 81, 82, 105
Fenugreek   24, 31, 36, 42, 43, 49, 57 - 59, 77, 78, 81, 96,
Fermented foods   25
Fig jam   32, 108
Frozen foods   25
Garam masala   31, 33, 43, 46, 79, 85
Garbanzo bean flour   24, 31, 33, 90, 93
Garlic cloves   24, 31, 33, 39, 42, 43, 57, 62, 75, 86, 87, 90, 97, 98, 100, 101, 104, 106, 107
Ghee   23-25, 31, 37-45, **47**, 53, 55, 57-64, 66, 67-70, 73, 74, 76-82, 85, 89-93, 95, 96, 98, 101, 102, 104-106, 108
Ginger   24, 31
    Crystallized   33, 73, 88
    Fresh   42, 50, 51, 59, 60, 64, 70, 72, 74, 76-79, 81-83, 96, 103, 105

Powder   37, 38, 40, 41, 46, 51, 54-56, 61, 66, 80, 93, 95
Goat chèvre   32, 85, 101
Great Northern Beans   32, 98
Gunas (Qualities)
    Physical   16, 27
    Subtle   17, 18, 27
Heavy whipping cream   32, 65
Honey   23, 32, 52, 69, 88
Jaggery   (see *Sugar*)
Kitcharis
    Calming Kitchari   43
    Chai Spice Kitchari with Fennel   60
    Womb Rejuvenating Kitchari   58
Lactation
    Breast milk   9, 13, 19, 25, 26, 28
    Teas
        Simple Lactation Tea   49
        Strong Fenugreek Tea   36
Lemon juice   24, 32, 39, 42, 57, 64, 75, 76, 84, 87, 88, 96, 100
Leftovers   25
Lime juice   24, 32, 88, 103, 107
Mama's Masala   43, 46, 57, 85
Maple syrup   24, 32, 36, 56, 73, 78, 82, 83, 92, 93, 98, 103
Meat   25
Milk   22 - 24, 31, 32
    Breast   (see *Lactation*)
    Coconut   56, 64, 72, 77-80, 105
    Dairy   38, 44, 50, 55, 66, 67, 68, 84
    Non-dairy   50, 52, 55, 61, 67, 68, 75, 80
Mint   20, 31, 103
Molasses   24, 32, 51, 61, 93, 95, 98
Mung   24, 31, 32
    Green whole mung beans   76
    Sprouted   32, 107
    Yellow split peeled mung dal   33, 42, 43, 58, 59, 60
Mushrooms   25
Nightshades   25
Nutmeg powder   24, 31, 40, 41, 45, 53, 55, 61, 64, 66, 70, 85

Oats   24, 31
   Flour   93
   Rolled   73
Ojas   23, 28
Paneer   24, **84**, 85, 101, 106-108 Pasta   26, 31
   Semolina (or Quinoa)   101
Pears   32, 56, 70
Pecans   31, 70, 88, 92, 108
Potatoes   *see Nightshades*
Pumpkin   32, 96 Quinoa   24, 31, 62, 101, 104
   Tasty Quinoa   62
Raisins   32, 51
Rasa   20
Raw foods   25
Rice   24, 31
   Basmati   37, 43, 53, 58, 60, 63, 67
   Cream of rice (farina)   41, 66
   Flour   93
   Noodles   107
   Simple Postpartum Rice   63
Rooibos (red tea)   31, 50
Saffron   23, 24, 31, 33, 44, 46, 54, 58, 61, 66, 68
Sesame seeds   24, 31, 46, 69, 86, 95, 100, 102
Sesame oil   24, 31, 37, 43, 55, 57-59, 63, 64, 73-76, 78, 81, 83, 85-87, 95-98, 100, 104, 107
Soups
   Black Bean Soup   97
   Butternut Squash Soup   64
   Creamy Beet Soup with Tarragon   75
   Healing Mung Soup   42
   Hearty Mung Bean Soup   76
   Hearty Roots & Barley Stew   74
   Mama's Mung Soup   59
   Replenishing Urad Dal Soup   57
   Toor Dal Soup with Pumpkin   96
Snacking Almonds   91
Spicy foods   25
Spinach   32, 77, 85, 101, 106
Strawberries   32, 72
Sugar   24, 32
   Coconut   33, 37, 40-42, 45, 55, 57, 59, 61, 66, 70, 73, 77, 95, 96, 102, 105, 107, 108
   Jaggery   33, 37, 45, 53, 70
   Turbinado   38, 44, 65, 67

Sugar snap peas   32, 107
Sweet potatoes   24, 32, 78, 80, 99, 106
Swiss chard   32, 78, 83
Tahini   31, 52, 100
Tamarind paste   24, 31, 33, 57, 59, 61, 102, 107
Tapioca   24, 31, 56
Tarragon   24, 31, 75
Tofu   32, 107
Tomatoes   *see Nightshades*
Toor dal   32, 33, 96
Turbinado cane sugar   (see *Sugar*)
Turmeric   24, 25, 31, 33, 37, 38, 42, 43, 57-60, 74, 76, 77, 79, 85, 96
Urad dal   24, 32, 33, 57
Vanilla   24, 31, 33, 53, 56, 65, 67, 72, 92
Vegetable Dishes
   Black Bean Croquets   104
   Curried Beets   79
   Curried Black Bean & Sweet Potato Burrito   106
   Delicious Yam Patties   102
   Garden Pasta with Pesto & Cheese   101
   Gingered Greens   83
   Glazed Carrots   82
   Happy Baby Fennel Dish   81
   Pesto Sweet Potato Fries   99
   Postnatal Pad Thai   107
   Sag Paneer   85
   Sweet Potato & Greens   78
   Sweet Potato Mash   80
   Vegetable Coconut Curry   77
   Vegetable Koorma with Fennel   105
Vipak   20
Virya   20
Whole wheat pastry flour   31, 89, 93, 108
Yams   24, 32, 68, 102
Yogurt   32, 108
Zucchini   32, 105

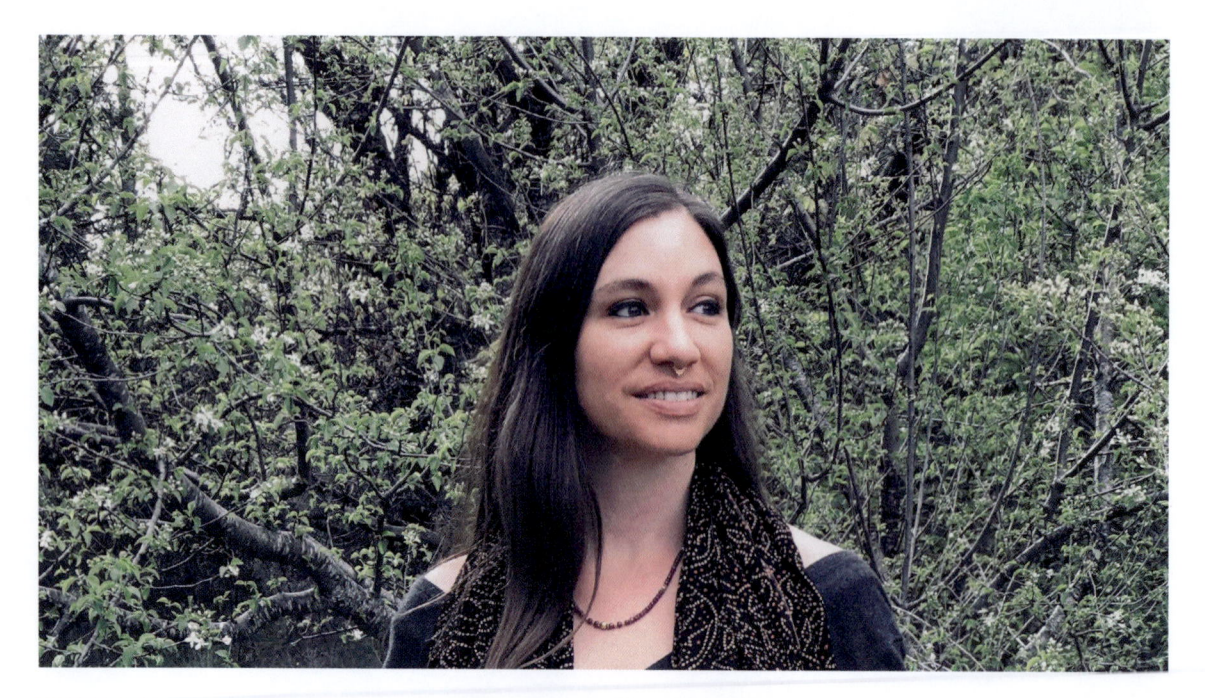

Ameya Duprey
BCTMB, NAMACB, AyurDoula

Ameya has been a vegetarian since the age of 15. Only when she began her formal training in Ayurveda 5 years later did she truly learn how to cook healthy and well-balanced vegetarian meals. Cooking delicious vegetarian food has been her passion for the last two decades.

In 2004, Ameya finished her Ayurvedic training with a focus on the cleansing and rejuvenating therapies of Pancha Karma. In 2011, she began specializing in the field of Ayurvedic postnatal care. She soon realized how essential an Ayurvedic postnatal diet was for the healing of both mother and breast-fed baby. She began sharing recipes and other knowledge on her blog ShaktiCare.com. Through the response from her blog, she came to realize the demand for a comprehensive cookbook for healing postpartum recipes.

Ameya lives with her husband and daughter in Northern California. She loves gardening, traveling the world, and eating chocolate, as well as practicing and performing the sacred Indian art of Odissi classical dance.

pinterest
@shakticare

facebook
@myshakticare

instagram
@shakticare

website
shakticare.com

Love Mama's Menu?

Take the next step to fully heal from birth with my FREE masterclass!

How to Fully Heal from Birth Without Feeling Stressed & Exhausted

Register at:
shakticare.com/masterclass

Printed in Great Britain
by Amazon